VOCATIONAL REHABILITATION

VOCATIONAL REHABILITATION

Jain Holmes MSc, Dip COT, OT

Chairperson COTSS in WORK
MJH Consultancy

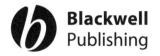
Blackwell
Publishing

Blackwell Publishing editorial offices:
Blackwell Publishing Ltd, 9600 Garsington Road, Oxford OX4 2DQ, UK
Tel: +44 (0)1865 776868
Blackwell Publishing Inc., 350 Main Street, Malden, MA 02148-5020, USA
Tel: +1 781 388 8250
Blackwell Publishing Asia Pty Ltd, 550 Swanston Street, Carlton, Victoria 3053, Australia
Tel: +61 (0)3 8359 1011

First published 2007 by Blackwell Publishing Ltd

ISBN: 978-1-4051-3364-7

Library of Congress Cataloging-in-Publication Data
Holmes, Jain.
Vocational rehabilitation / Jain Holmes.
p. ; cm.
Includes bibliographical references and index.
ISBN-13: 978-1-4051-3364-7 (pbk. : alk. paper)
1. Vocational rehabilitation. I. Title.
[DNLM: 1. Rehabilitation, Vocational–Great Britain.   HD 7256.G7 H749v 2007]
HD7255.H65 2007
362.4′0484–dc22
2007013129

A catalogue record for this title is available from the British Library

Set in 10/12.5pt Sabon
by Graphicraft Limited, Hong Kong
Printed and bound in Singapore
by Fabulous Printers Pte Ltd

The publisher's policy is to use permanent paper from mills that operate a sustainable forestry
policy, and which has been manufactured from pulp processed using acid-free and elementary
chlorine-free practices. Furthermore, the publisher ensures that the text paper and cover board used
have met acceptable environmental accreditation standards.

For further information on Blackwell Publishing, visit our website:
www.blackwellpublishing.com

Cover photographic image © Christian Lagerek – FOTOLIA

CONTENTS

PREFACE

Vocational rehabilitation is a topic of increasing popularity in the UK among businesses, the government, the voluntary and charity sector, the insurance sector, the unions and healthcare organisations. This increase in attention to facilitating people into work is driven politically to reduce the heavy bill on the then Incapacity Benefit (now the Employment Support Allowance). There is also an improved understanding of the benefits of work for many people and an awareness that common health problems should not necessarily lead to long-term sickness absence or job loss. Many practitioners from a range of agencies recognise this, understand how long-term sickness can result in chronic ill health and are experienced in rehabilitation and facilitation techniques to address issues of reduced function, loss of confidence and low self-efficacy that accompany long term sickness absence from work.

While there is an abundance of information about vocational rehabilitation, sickness absence and employment support, there remains a paucity of evidence about which interventions really work in vocational rehabilitation. Also there is limited information and sound research data on which designs of vocational services achieve the outcomes they set out to or how they achieve their outcomes. There is growing evidence for the Individual Placement and Support Model, a type of supported employment, with measures produced to indicate how closely a service is meeting the model's parameters – but more of this is required for the other models and interventions. This information is very relevant to practitioners working in modern locations that are providing or might potentially provide vocational services and in the competitive and complicated world of work in the 21st century. There is an increasing array of guidance from government departments that focus on vocational rehabilitation:

- A variety of National Service Frameworks from the Department of Health
- Guidance for commissioners about commissioning vocational rehabilitation services
- Guidance from the Health and Safety Executive about sickness absence and return to work
- The Vocational Rehabilitation Framework from the Department of Work and Pensions

These are helpful and informative documents encouraging practitioners, employers and service users to engage with vocational rehabilitation and to facilitate the potential that people have in achieving their own goals for work in whatever way suits best. However, on the whole these documents do not provide the nitty-gritty detail about what to do – they are not manuals for vocational rehabilitation. There are also quite a number of books already written about vocational rehabilitation, but the majority have been written for practitioners in countries other than the UK. Simultaneous to the emerging interest in supporting people to return to work is an emergence of vocational rehabilitation services. However, practitioners supporting people to return to work and open employment do not have an abundance of manuals or culturally relevant texts (yet) to assist them design vocationally relevant rehabilitation programmes for the 21st century.

The aim of this book is to provide some guidance to practitioners involved in vocational rehabilitation. It aims to explain vocational rehabilitation as it is in the UK at the time of writing and to explain a range of relevant interventions for vocational rehabilitation services in the UK. It aims to be a source of information of good practice for practitioners currently providing return to work services as well as those intending to develop services.

I want to emphasise that the perspective for this text is practitioner based and as I am an occupational therapist, it is important to recognise that my professional philosophies and as such my emphases on issues will reflect my professional background. That said, one of the greatest experiences I have had while writing this book has been to learn about how other people, including other practitioners, employers and clients, perceive vocational rehabilitation and potential pathways for returning to work.

The intended readership for this book is the practitioner interested in facilitating people to return to work. They may include occupational therapists, physiotherapists, psychologists and psychotherapists. It may also be of interest to occupational health nurses, human resource departments, occupational health physicians, GPs and employment support practitioners. It could be suitable for pre- and post-registration students studying vocational rehabilitation.

The evidence contained within this book comes from many sources and where possible I have cited these so that readers can have the opportunity to make their own minds up on issues raised herein. It is not my intention to give full academic arguments for each point that is raised, as other authors write these eloquently in research-based publications. I have attempted to systematically appraise the evidence before presenting it in this book and where possible any recommendations that are made are specifically linked to supporting evidence. However, as Paula Hyde (2004) indicates, there is no gold standard of evidence, it just depends what your question is. So the types of evidence that have been used have depended on the questions I was asking.

This book cannot address all aspects of vocational rehabilitation with all client groups and so it will primarily have a focus on vocational rehabilitation into the open employment market. It will aim to cover a range of disabilities and health reasons for being off sick from work but not focus on impairments, as these do not necessarily indicate the difficulties people have in the work context. Other texts are currently being written that will address severe mental health issues particularly and specifically occupational therapy in vocational rehabilitation.

The five chapters cover the pathways that an individual may take in returning to work after a period of being off sick from work. Chapter 1 introduces vocational rehabilitation, suggesting some definitions and setting it in the context of the UK. This section introduces some of the range of services that might be included as vocational rehabilitation.

Chapter 2 addresses three assessment strategies – person-based assessments, the environment-based assessments and the assessment of function in relation to work.

Chapter 3 looks at what can be done with the results of assessments and suggests how to problem solve and analyse the assessment data and then develop appropriate goals.

Chapter 4 relates to the potentially vast array of interventions within vocational rehabilitation and covers the statutory, private, independent and voluntary sectors. It also raises issues about evidence-based practice and practical issues relating to a vocational rehabilitation programme. This chapter covers three types of intervention: those related to health and social care; those related to career choice and career decision-making; and workplace-related interventions.

Chapter 5 is about establishing a vocational rehabilitation service and looks at considerations around the topics of funding a programme, location of a facility, staff mix, marketing, sources of referrals and outcome measurement. It also describes briefly some of the contemporary projects in a range of vocational rehabilitation providers.

This book has, for me, been both a pleasure and a huge commitment to put into practice. I hope that you will find it useful and easy to read and that you get a sense of my enthusiasm for the field of vocational rehabilitation. There is nothing more satisfying to me as an occupational therapist than to empower someone to be able to go out and feel they have done a good day's work.

The Peak District, Derbyshire, May 2007 *JAH*

Reference

Hyde P (2004) Fool's Gold: Examining the use of gold standards in the production of research evidence. *British Journal of Occupational Therapy* 67(2): 89–94.

ACKNOWLEDGEMENTS

This book has been a most interesting journey for me, taking me to places that I never experienced before. Of course I don't mean that I have been away to foreign parts discovering new and fantastic ways of helping people back to work – I only need to travel around the UK to see great projects and fantastic practitioners. The journey for me has been one of self-discovery. Never in my secondary school days did I think I could ever be clever enough to write a book and to think that other people might read what I had written was only something that other (clever) people achieved. However, my lecturers at occupational therapy school inspired me with enthusiasm for the work I was in training to do and this enthusiasm has stayed with me ever since, so thank you all at what was St Andrew's School of Occupational Therapy between 1987 and 1990.

I love teaching people about new ideas and new ways of doing things and to experience somebody picking up a new skill, or enveloping new knowledge is wonderful. It must be a family trait as my *Seanair* (Grandad in Gaelic) was a teacher as are other members of my family and my aunt who is an occupational therapist in Scotland introduced to me the profession of occupational therapy – in many ways a profession about imparting functional skills. It doesn't matter whether it is my clients, my colleagues or the students I see, the feeling of fulfilment when they realise they can do something they couldn't before, or they understand a concept which is new to them is humbling. This book for me is another way of passing on information.

The information in this book is not just my own set of ideas but a coming together of conversations and debates I have had with clients and colleagues over the past few years, the grasping of new and sometimes challenging ideas I had not encountered before, and the reading of published and unpublished work by other people also passionate about helping people to achieve their occupational aspirations. Without all the interactions with these people, I wouldn't have been able to put down on paper what I have done. So thank you.

I need to pay special thanks to those colleagues who have painstakingly looked at my work and critiqued it and offered advice to me. So thank you to Heather Watson, Julie Leeson, Liz Howsley, Deborah Unwin and Kay Orr.

I want to say a huge thank-you to my mum who checked every chapter in this book for spelling, grammar and comprehension. This was a huge piece of work for her to do and fit into her very busy schedule. Thank-you mum. Finally, thank you to my husband and young children for putting up with me working ridiculous hours and being less than the domestic goddess they were used to!

I know all these acknowledgments won't mean much to most people, but all of the people mentioned and alluded to here have actually been the reason that this book has been completed.

ABBREVIATIONS

ASSET	assessment, employment and training
AtW	access to work
BTE	Baltimore therapeutic equipment
CBT	cognitive behavioural therapy
CIC	community interest company
CMP	condition management programmes
COPM	Canadian Occupational Performance Measure
DASH	disabilities of the arm, shoulder and hand
DAT	disability advisory team
DDA	Disability Discrimination Act
DNA	did not attend
DOT	Dictionary of Occupational Titles
DPQ	Dallas Pain Questionnaire
DRO	disablement resettlement officer
DSE	display screen equipment
EAP	employee assistance programme
ELCI	employers' liability compulsory insurance
EPP	expert patients programme
EQRM	European Quality in Rehabilitation Mark
ERC	employment rehabilitation centre
ESA	Employment and Support Allowance
FCE	functional capacity evaluation
GP	general practitioner
IB	incapacity benefit
IBPA	incapacity benefit personal advisor
ICF	International Classification of Functioning, Disability and Health
IPS	individual placement and support
JIA	juvenile idiopathic arthritis
JRRP	job retention and rehabilitation pilot
METs	metabolic equivalents of oxygen consumption
MODAPTS	modular arrangement for predetermined time standards
MOHO	model of human occupation
MTM	Methods Time Measurement
NDDP	New Deal for Disabled People
NDI	Neck Disability Index
NVQ	National Vocational Qualification
OHS	occupational health service

PACT	placing, assessment and counselling team
PAS	personal assistance services
PCP	person-centred planning
PCT	primary care trust
PMTS	predetermined motion time system
PPE	personal protective equipment
RTW	return to work
SCCT	social cognitive career theory
SCQF	Scottish Credit and Qualifications Framework
SDS	self-directed search
SOAP	subjective–objective–analysis–plan
SWOT	strengths-weaknesses-opportunities-threats
USA	United States of America
VCWS	Valpar Component Work Samples
WEIS	Work Environment Impact Scale
WIS	Work Instability Scale
WRI	Worker Role Interview

Chapter 1
INTRODUCING VOCATIONAL REHABILITATION

Introduction

This chapter explains the context of vocational rehabilitation, describes a continuum of support for people engaging in work and looks at the semantics surrounding work and vocational rehabilitation. It will also explore some of the international comparisons of vocational rehabilitation and whether any of the practices elsewhere can be applied to the UK and – more importantly – to the setting in which you work. Finally, this chapter will briefly describe the importance of holistic assessments, the importance of goal setting, what might be construed as vocational rehabilitation, who provides the service and where the services might be found in the UK.

History of vocational rehabilitation

'It (work) is deeply embedded in a political–economic–societal context that nudges and constrains the translation of technology into work activities and people's participation in them.' (Howard 1995)

This is an important concept to grasp, as it helps to explain the changes in work over time and inevitably, therefore, the kind of work activities that will form part of vocational rehabilitation. The history of interventions that focused on work and the emergence of occupational therapy is somewhat intertwined. Paterson in Pratt and Jacobs 199 also says that this emergence relates to

'complex sociological, political, economic and technological factors.'

Early 20th century

There is a 200-year history of the explicit use of occupation in the rehabilitation of people with both psychological (then called insanity) and physical problems (then the common infectious diseases, especially tuberculosis). In about 1917, the people who had started using occupation as a 'cure' also founded occupational therapy in the USA. In the UK, Dr Elizabeth Casson founded occupational therapy after visiting the Boston School of Occupational Therapy and she set up an Occupational Therapy course in 1929. She also set up the Allendale Curative Workshop in 1939, which was an outpatient department for people suffering from physical disease or disability (Pratt & Jacobs 1997). Occupational therapy texts that were written in the early days always focused on returning the client to work using the grading of activities.

Both World Wars were instrumental in pushing the boundaries in industry and making developments in technology, medicine and thus in rehabilitation. Around the World Wars developed the emerging concepts that we now understand as ergonomics and fitting the task to the man; and there was greater urgency to assist people injured in the Second World War to return to work to support the economy.

Post-war

In 1944 in the UK the Disabled Persons Act came into being as a result of the need for large numbers of injured soldiers returning from the Second World War to get back into work. The Disabled Persons Act 1944 brought in four ways of helping disabled people:

- Quota system
- Industrial rehabilitation units
- Resettlement service
- Sheltered workshops

Between 1944 and 1995, no other legislation was introduced that would affect the way in which people would be rehabilitated back into work (Floyd 1997). Vocational rehabilitation after the war might not be recognised as the range of models seen today as it was more closely related to what is now known as sheltered employment (Curtis online). Since 1948 there have been many social changes – some of these have been highlighted by Waddell and Aylward (2005):

- Economic prosperity and rising material standards of living
- Labour market changes and patterns of work (globalisation, greater flexibility and mobility, more part-time and fixed contract working, lower job security)
- The role of women and family structures (in particular the number of women working, gender equality issues and lone parent families) and increasing female participation in the labour market
- Patterns of retirement (increased life expectancy, increased availability of employment pensions, trends to early retirement, working fewer years but living longer in retirement)
- Attitudes to work, sickness, disability and social security benefits
- Individual liberty and rising expectations
- Disenchantment with state and professional authority

As early as 1913 in the USA, an occupational therapy leader, Herbert Hall, saw the role of the hospital expanding to include vocational training. He suggested to the Massachusetts General Hospital in Boston that they open up a 'workshop' that patients would use after being discharged from hospital but before they were ready to return to work. In 1920 in the USA, the Vocational Rehabilitation Act was passed and the foundations for vocational rehabilitation were started (Cromwell 1985).

The National Health Service (NHS) hospitals' rehabilitation departments were often found providing work/vocational rehabilitation, especially in the occupational therapy department. Following discharge from hospital, the patient would be referred to the occupational therapy outpatient department for further rehabilitation to improve tolerances to activities. They would also likely be referred to other outpatient departments too, but it was the occupational therapy department that would house the workshops. Quite often there would be a workshop or several workshops where a patient would start off at the light end of the workshop, gradually moving towards the 'heavy' end – after which it was determined at some point that discharge from the service was imminent. The workshops were set up to replicate different kinds of work tasks, using equipment such as treadle saws, hand-operated drilling machines and lathes. All student occupational therapists were trained how to use these kinds of machines in their basic training (as I did in the late 1980s).

Patients (as the service users were commonly called then) had rehabilitation programmes designed for them by the occupational therapist to improve physical and psychological tolerances to increasingly harder activities. This was to prepare people for managing at work and managing the maintenance-type tasks in the home. Technical staff supervised patients on a daily basis with the occupational therapist reviewing the programmes and arranging with the technician how to grade the machines and tasks to continue rehabilitation.

Workplace visits would occur occasionally, with negotiations taking place with workplace managers to organise return to work plans. Another referral point at this stage was the Disablement Resettlement Officer (DRO) at the Job Centre, previously the Ministry of Labour Office (Floyd 1997). The DRO could arrange the registration of the individual to be named as 'disabled' and they could refer individuals on to the employment (previously industrial) rehabilitation centres (ERC) that were available in most cities after the 1950s. At the ERC, an individual would be given a week's assessment and then a rehabilitation programme to help them back into employment. Individuals would be seen by unit occupational therapists and occupational psychologists and this would involve skills training, career decision making as well as job searching. At first, these ERCs had a success rate of 75% for returning people to work in open employment (Floyd 1997; Curtis online).

It was already recognised that not everyone would be suited to open employment and sheltered workshops were used to give disabled people the chance to earn money (not necessarily at the market rate) in a secure and supportive environment. Remploy was the Government-established organisation to provide sheltered work and some local authorities and charities also developed these services. In the 1980s and 1990s the sheltered employment model was dying out as being appropriate for everyone and being replaced with alternatives such as support in open employment. The WORKSTEP scheme was the closest relation to what was understood by sheltered workshops (Curtis online).

Late 20th century

By the mid 1970s the outcomes for people obtaining open employment in the ERCs had dropped to below 50%. A review of the system found that the arrangement was outdated (Floyd 1997) and out of the closure of the rehabilitation centres came:

- Fewer but more effective Assessment, Employment and Training (ASSET) centres with newer assessment methods
- Jobcentres offering financial help for employers in the first few weeks of work (now the job introduction scheme)
- The current Access to Work scheme that assisted with:
  - Fares to work
  - Advice and financial assistance to reduce workplace barriers
  - Personal assistants for some work duties

Following reorganisations, the DRO was replaced by the Disability Advisory Team and in the 1990s by the PACT – Placing, Assessment and Counselling Team. With the closure of the ERCs the nearest scheme today is 'work preparation' delivered by the voluntary sector and commissioned through the Jobcentre Plus (Curtis online).

With the reorganisation of the NHS when trust status was developed in the early 1990s there came a heightened awareness of affording the services that were being delivered. The perceived issues with the occupational therapy workshops were that they did not reflect the current business of the acute hospital and that they were perhaps superfluous and a luxury. Many of the workshops disappeared in the hospitals but the valuable aims they achieved were never replaced. In my lifetime as an occupational therapist, I have seen workshop after workshop close down, the space used for other purposes and the focus of 'work' and vocational rehabilitation lost. There remain some valuable workshops in some UK hospitals, but they and their technicians are, on the whole, a rare breed. So the NHS hospitals' core business was acute healthcare, not work; and NHS community services' core business was longer-term healthcare of those who could not work; and social services' core business was social care. But no one was taking real responsibility for vocational rehabilitation, so gradually, vocational rehabilitation has been eroded from occupational therapy departments and preregistration training in universities.

Renewed vision

The good news is that now the Government sees the benefits of return to work rehabilitation and support in a renewed vision and so the push is on again to revive vocational rehabilitation across the country in a contemporary framework.

Undergraduate courses are starting to include work as a key element to their students' studies and now it is not just the domain of the occupational therapist or the occupational psychologist. The emphasis is interdisciplinary and multiagency education.

How has your service approach developed over time?

How does your service link with other agencies and professions?

Driving UK vocational rehabilitation

Politics and the Government have a great influence over health services and work as already indicated (Howard 1995; Floyd 1997; Pratt & Jacobs 1997; Curtis online). Government affects how supply and demand for services work because there is a constant need to constantly the flow of money for the entire country. Put simply, the Government has to have sufficient money coming in to the country to spend on all the key areas (education, health, etc.). The current issues of an ageing population and decreasing birth rate gives rise to concern about the numbers of potential workers available in the population to achieve the desired economic activity for the Treasury. So it has become important for the Government to look at who is not working in the UK at any one time and develop ways to enable them to become economically active.

However, while the inactive population in the 1940s were demobbed and injured military personnel, the contemporary picture is quite different. This requires a different approach to the 1940s solutions. The social benefits paid to disabled people increased significantly between 1970 and 1990; and unemployment rates have also risen. The proportion of disabled people unemployed is much larger when compared with able-bodied people and statistics indicate that in the region of 20% of the total number of disabled people are unemployed. This compares with less than 10% of able-bodied people (Floyd & Barrett 2005). The numbers are somewhat academic in the context of this book, but the reason for mentioning them here is to show the vast difference in the proportions. The Government monitors the numbers of people claiming different social benefits, those unemployed and those who say they would like to be able to work. These statistics go some way to influencing policies, together with a changing social consciousness about how to improve the well-being of everyone.

Legislation

There are numerous pieces of legislation that relate to either employment, health or welfare benefits, which all impact on how vocational rehabilitation services are designed, operate and are commissioned.

Building Capacity for Work: A UK Framework for Vocational Rehabilitation (Department for Work and Pensions (DWP) 2004a): Explains the drivers for vocational rehabilitation and related Government initiatives.

Disability Discrimination Act (DDA) 1995: The most influential piece of legislation to affect the vocational rehabilitation field in recent times is the Disability Discrimination Act 1995 (Floyd 2002); together with the establishment of the Disability Rights Commission to help implement the DDA.

'It reflects a growing awareness of the need to provide disabled people with support in all forms of employment, rather than just focusing on help with finding employment as was the case in the past.' (Floyd 2002)

The DWP (2004a) says:

'The drivers include statistics that show that, although there has been no worsening of health in the UK since the early 1980s, labour market participation and sickness absence remains an issue.'

Employers Liability Compulsory Insurance Review (DWP 2003): This stated the Government's commitment to produce the vocational rehabilitation framework for the UK and also highlighted that rehabilitation is at the heart of the response to injury and ill-health (DWP 2004b).

A Strategy for Workplace Health and Safety in Great Britain to 2010 (HSC 2004): This Health and Safety Commission (HSC) publication looks at increasing the role that health and safety takes in strategies for return to work and sickness absence management. The job retention and rehabilitation pilots between 2003 and 2005 were a joint initiative between the DWP, Department of Health (DH) and the Health and Safety Executive (HSE) and was a randomised controlled trial designed to test the

'net impact of a person-centred case management approach.'(DWP 2004)

Choosing Health: Making Healthier Choices Easier (DH 2004): This was a joint strategy document between the DWP, DH and HSE in 2005. It looks at bringing together all the valuable work currently being undertaken inside and outside Government. The first National Director for Health and Work was appointed as a result of this and the Director will have a role in promoting and improving health in the workplace (www.health-and-work.gov.uk).

I considered stating lots of statistics to illustrate the nature of the issues facing the British population regarding disability, work, health and well-being but I have deliberately left these out – partly because they date so quickly and partly because they can be interpreted sometimes in the eye of the beholder. There are no statistics related to contemporary vocational rehabilitation programmes, for instance how many programmes there are in different sectors, how many practitioners work in these settings and whether vocational rehabilitation is the primary goal of their interventions or secondary to other roles. I hope that in the future there will be meaningful statistics to report.

The essence of work

Adolph Meyer in 1977 wrote that healthy living involved a 'blending of work and pleasure.' (Cromwell 1985)

Work can be defined in many ways and has different meanings for different people. It covers the following descriptions:

- Physical, mental effort directed towards doing or making something
- Paid employment
- A duty, task
- The place, office where someone works
- To handle or manipulate
- To make one's way with effort
- Productive activity
- It is an expression of what people are, it is human purpose (Collins Concise Dictionary 1989)

Work is a major part of most people's lives and provides the income by which people can sustain life, independence and security. Work provides structure to everyday life and the social contact and the status that helps to define the person in his or her environment and in society. Participation in work is one of the major routes to social inclusion, which then provides some dignity and the opportunity to contribute to society (Waddell & Aylward 2005).

Work has been shown to have good effects on physical and mental well-being in terms of (Waddell & Aylward 2005):

- Symptom management
- Recovery and rehabilitation
- Self-esteem and confidence
- Social identity and role
- Normalisation of activities and participation
- Improved social functioning
- Quality of life
- Social inclusion

Work and return to work used to be part of rehabilitation in the NHS and remain so in some parts of the UK. However, the focus of rehabilitation to return to work is no longer a high priority focus of British healthcare. With the positive effects on well-being, it seems reasonable to consider that vocational rehabilitation, including job retention and return to work, should be the ultimate goals and outcomes for healthcare providers, rehabilitation providers and the social security system (Waddell & Aylward 2005).

Being out of work can have negative effects on people's well-being and these have summarised by Waddell and Aylward (2005) as:

- Loss of fitness
- Physical and mental deterioration
- Poor physical and mental health
- Psychological distress and depression
- Loss of work related habits and attitudes
- Increased suicide and mortality rates
- Poverty
- Social exclusion

What effects do working and not working have on your clients?

How would you cope if you were off sick for weeks at a time?

Social exclusion

'happens when people or places suffer from a series of problems such as unemployment, discrimination, poor skills, low incomes, poor housing, high crime, ill health and family breakdown. When such problems combine they can create a vicious cycle.' (www.socialexclusionunit.gov.uk)

Palmer et al. (2006) say:

'Working-age disability is widespread and its link to low income clear-cut.'

There has been an increase in long-term illness and disability recorded and the challenge now is to support disabled people through a variety of methods into work (Stanley in Roulstone & Barnes 2005). It is seen that enabling disabled people to engage with work will reduce their social exclusion, but does that work have to be paid to improve social inclusion? Or is there room to debate the worthwhile economic and social contributions that people can make outside the paid employment arena? It is suggested by some that the ablist attitudes link too much disability with inability (Barnes 1991 in Roulstone & Barnes 2005). There is no scope to explore social exclusion in depth here, but it is recognised that this is an important topic to investigate further.

The world of work is in a state of flux as indicated by Howard (1995) with an

'increasing number of flexible employers who use casual labour and of flexible workers who are engaged in flexitime or home-based work.' (Steward 1997)

Some employers will themselves provide flexible patterns of work for employees. Using concepts such as flexi-hours allows greater control over the work environment by the employee. New technology and teleworking reduces the need to travel into a workplace with reduced conformity to particular codes of dress or other traditional work behaviours that may be required in a place of work.

'Aided by new computer and communications technology, the management, development and clerical staff can work away from the core office, in satellite offices in cheaper suburban areas or at home.' (Steward 1997)

The flexibility in hours and place of work will, for some people, encourage better control over balancing work and home commitments and open up the potential to work. Women who traditionally stayed at home to provide childcare, and single-parent families who may have no choice but to stay at home may now be able to tap into potential work from home. For example, some people are already using online auction sites to set up small enterprises to earn money by trading in a variety of commodities. Being at home and working can still offer the opportunity of social contact if the home worker decides to take on staff as business grows. Vocational rehabilitation should be able to reflect these changes by looking at everything the world of work can offer clients with a wide range of working needs.

Changes in the world of work can also have negative consequences potentially.

'As traditional waged work decreases, contract work will be tendered with targets and deadlines that suit the customers, not the workers.' (Steward 1997)

In an increasingly competitive and global market, often the cheapest labour costs win over the more expensive; faster completion times win over slower ones; and organisations with higher numbers of people returning to work may win over those achieving fewer numbers of clients returning to work. But cheaper, faster and more numbers does not necessarily mean better working conditions for workers or better quality results at the end of the day. Vocational rehabilitation services may be contracted to achieve quotas of service users to return to work in the short term, with little chance to show the quality of work placements or the long-term (longer than three months or a year) sustainability and long tenure of people in work.

Increasing productivity rates and flexible working times may mean that unsocial hours are unrecognised, forcing workers to complete targets over 24-hour periods rather than recognising that work stops at six o'clock. This pressure to achieve outcomes at all costs will never sit comfortably with many people. Home working is seen as a flexible alternative for some people – but it will not suit everyone. Some people may become even more isolated working from home. For others, this could be a distinct advantage and the understanding of social behaviour and social interactions may be more manageable without face-to-face contact. Working from a home environment that has already been adapted could be easier to manage than 'making do' in another work environment that may have physical accessibility problems, or a culture of negative attitudes towards sickness absence and disability.

Describing vocational rehabilitation

Rehabilitation is defined using the World Health Organization's descriptions made in 1974 as

'the combined and coordinated use of medical, social, educational and vocational measures for training or retraining the individual to the highest possible level of functional ability.' (WHO 1974)

Hagedorn (2000) explains that rehabilitation

'is a deliberately structured therapeutic process.'

The concept of rehabilitation has been around since shortly after World War One when veterans needed some way of reintegrating into the working world again.

Defining vocational rehabilitation is a topic often hotly debated in the UK, as are many other semantic issues. What meaning one derives from a word is often based on one's own experiences and fundamental beliefs about the world. So vocational rehabilitation seems to mean a wide range of things here in the UK. In fact 'vocational' in the 1970s was deliberately not used in the naming of the ERCs because it was commonly associated with taking a vocation in the church or the law and would convey the wrong meaning (Curtis online). This debate does not seem as prevalent in other countries where vocational rehabilitation services are established and structured and where legislation and Government welfare is explicitly entwined with work and return to work.

The question seems to raise many issues about how one interprets the words vocational and rehabilitation. Does 'vocational' mean 'work'? Does it mean 'employment'? Does it mean 'productive engagement in activity'? Does 'rehabilitation' pertain to health issues, to psychological issues, to criminal activity, to social issues? *Building Capacity for Work: A UK Framework for Vocational Rehabilitation* (DWP 2004a) states that the DWP work

'highlighted that the term vocational rehabilitation means different things to different stakeholders.'

The report goes on to suggest that until services are more established, this working description of vocational rehabilitation is used:

'Vocational rehabilitation is a process to overcome the barriers an individual faces when accessing, remaining or returning to work following injury, illness or impairment. This process includes the procedures in place to support the individual and/or employer or others (e.g. family and carers), including help to access vocational rehabilitation and to practically manage the delivery of vocational rehabilitation.' (DWP 2004a)

For the purposes of this book this working description will be used to under-pin the concepts and descriptions. Vocational rehabilitation is representative of a wide range of vocational and educational services that are offered to people who are working, as well as those out of work or who have never worked. These services are designed to help an individual choose a vocational direction and determine the course needed to achieve the chosen goal. Interventions to achieve an occupational goal. may include

'*an assessment of needs, retraining and capacity building, return to work management by employers, reasonable adjustments and control measures, disability awareness, condition management and medical treatment*' (DWP 2004a)

International comparisons

It would be fair to say that other countries as well as our own have influenced contemporary vocational rehabilitation in the UK. As the USA has had a Vocational Rehabilitation Act since the 1920s, it is hardly surprising that they have a wealth of information that can be accessed. However, directly transposing overseas programmes may not necessarily fit the UK culture, health and social care systems and welfare benefits.

North America: The North American countries are excellent at producing systematic protocols for assessments, vocational guidance and work preparation. This has been helped by their extensive databases about occupational information, which describe the functional demands of jobs and the training required to pursue the career choice. The USA has also developed the concept of supported employment and this is now the favoured approach over sheltered employment. This seems to have developed as greater understanding of the societal barriers to return to work have been recognised. The notion now is to place and train rather than to train and place (Floyd 2002; Godby 2005). The Individual Placement and Support (IPS) programmes are recommended and are producing significant evidence and outcome measurement (Floyd 2002; DH 2006;).

Scandinavia: The Scandinavian countries are prolific producers of evidence related to job retention and multidisciplinary team approaches to return to work and are based on similar healthcare and social systems to the UK.

Australasia: Australasia has developed the vocational rehabilitation profession many years ago with the development of the Rehabilitation Counselling Association of Australia (www.rcaa.org.au), which demonstrates the requirement for carefully trained staff, monitored through standards of practice and accountable to an overall registration body. From a variety of countries has come and flourished the case management approach that has become important in the overall co-ordination of individuals' rehabilitation and return to work.

The UK contribution to vocational rehabilitation is built mostly on valuable localised initiatives that have been dependent on individuals, local interest and expertise (Godby 2005). These initiatives have produced useful and practical applications of vocational rehabilitation in particular sectors and with particular groups of people. Possibly the largest advances being made are in the field of mental health, culminating in the publication of guidance for the NHS commissioners – *Vocational Services for People with Severe Mental Health Problems* (DH 2006).

What does vocational rehabilitation look like today?

When people engage with rehabilitation there is a perception that something is being done to them to remedy a particular problem or issue. When vocational rehabilitation is mentioned, it is interesting to consider what is actually meant by this term. To some people it could mean help with returning to a job, to others it could mean training to obtain a job, to others it doesn't relate to jobs at all but to meaningful occupation, voluntary work or engagement in activity that is purposeful. Waddell et al. (2004) say that rehabilitation must focus on

'identifying and overcoming the health, personal/psychological, and social/ occupational obstacles to recovery and (return to) work.'

Vocational rehabilitation seems to reflect a variety of interventions today that span a range of options including meaningful occupations through:

- Voluntary work
- Sheltered work
- Supported employment
- Open employment opportunities

An individual should be able to access different options at different times of their life depending on their needs at a particular point in time. Moving from paid employment into voluntary work should not come with the common attitude that it is an easier option than open employment. Sheltered work and meaningful occupations should not be seen as the lowest aspirations for people, with only those reaching paid employment on the open market attaining the pinnacle of achievement.

The Trades Union Congress (TUC) (2006b) says that it is important to remove the inequality that remains in workplaces including systematic discrimination, attitudes and practices, inaccessible workplaces and equipment. The TUC also identify other barriers such as housing, education and transport as being key to improving the difficulties that many disabled people face when trying to compete on equal terms in the open labour market.

The TUC has a three-point plan in place, which is aimed at helping disabled people into employment:

1. Prevention of people leaving the workforce through designing-out problems.
2. Retention of staff with every employer having to draw up a return to work plan during an employee's sick leave.

3. Interventions in the form of nationally available programmes such as the roll out of Pathways to Work. with help continuing after clients have moved into employment. (www.tuc.org.uk)

Modern vocational rehabilitation perhaps needs to take account of prevention work as well as job retention work and return to work, as the TUC suggests. Many of the vocational rehabilitation practitioners I meet are battling with their managers to initiate services that will address their client's work needs in a meaningful way. The rehabilitation staff of the NHS are in the main hungry for training about helping their clients to work – whatever the personal meaning of the word. Modern vocational rehabilitation should not be about trying to fit people into pigeonholes of services just to meet the outcome requirements of funding. It should be individualised intervention that is led by the service user, with the service making changes to engage fully with its clients. If there is a service user who is not following 'the programme' then it is surely up to the service to change to meet the client's needs, and not the client who necessarily has to change. The change might not involve altering the whole programme, but looking at attitudes about missed appointments, looking beyond the lost time to finding out what has precipitated the 'DNA' (did not attend). Motivational issues should be part and parcel of the vocational rehabilitation programme, as should self-efficacy. One without the other misses important areas of need in a person.

It is not enough to provide job searching or assessment facilities without understanding the service user and providing a long-term commitment to help them find sustainable work. There seems very little merit in helping someone to return to work if they are then left to return to the cycle of downward-spiralling function. Some people will only need a few signposts to put them on the right track to return to work and perhaps this is where future research should focus. Exploring whether it is possible to determine the likelihood of a person needing lots of assistance could be helpful in developing services and resources. If this kind of determination could be made at the earliest point of illness or injury, then the employer or GP could help to signpost people to the right service locally. Contemporary services remain patchy and difficult to map, difficult to refer to (because they are difficult to find) and there is no measure yet of whether the service you find is actually delivering what they say are delivering.

What can be involved in a programme?

The programme should match the needs of the individual with the needs of the workplace. This is independent of whether the person is in paid employment, voluntary work, sheltered work or work-type tasks (i.e. tasks that are purposeful but occur in a defined setting, such as a long-term care unit or at home). Figure 1.1 outlines what might be considered in a vocational rehabilitation programme. It has been adapted from Roy Matheson's (2004) original diagram, developed as teaching materials for students learning about functional capacity evaluations.

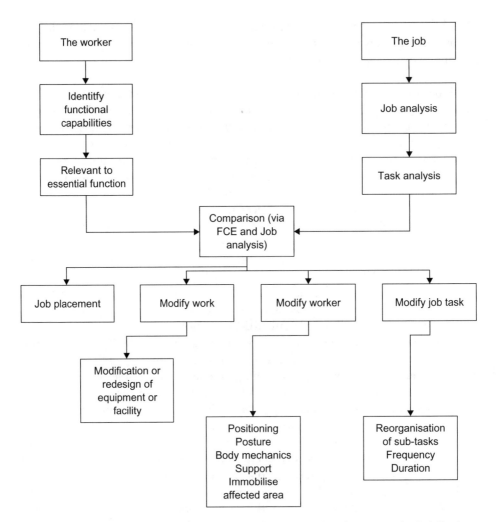

Figure 1.1 Outline of the potential interventions associated with vocational rehabilitation.

However, there are many other potential services that might be included in vocational rehabilitation – such as training and education, career counselling and job brokering.

It will not be possible in this book to cover all of these potential services, describe them and do justice to them. However, they may be mentioned throughout the text and then defined in the glossary. Remember that if someone defines a service by a particular term, such as job broker, you will still need to explore what it provides by speaking with them or looking at their website.

For the purposes of this book, we will concentrate on those services that will assist people to return to paid or voluntary work and will therefore not include training and education in broad abilities such as life skills, communication skills and social skills (also considered prevocational skills).

Who can be involved in delivering vocational rehabilitation?

Chapter 5 addresses the various stakeholders in vocational rehabilitation and these can be seen in Table 5.2. Potential providers of vocational rehabilitation are somewhat difficult to determine at this fast-developing stage of the profession. However, it is quite likely that the following agencies will be involved with provision if they are not already involved:

- Employee self-help groups
- Expert patients
- Primary care trusts (PCTs)
- Some secondary care in the NHS
- Local authorities
- Voluntary and charity organisations
- Occupational health services
- Independent businesses and practitioners
- Trades unions
- Employers
- Government programmes
- Health and Safety Executive programmes
- Insurance industry
- Education sector

As is mentioned later in the book, there is no regulation of vocational rehabilitation providers under one umbrella. Health professionals will be regulated under their own regulatory body such as the Health Professions Council, other practitioners may sign up to the ethical standards of certain bodies, but there are no standards set down for vocational rehabilitation and it is the push of organisations such as the vocational rehabilitation association (www.vocationalrehabilitationassociation.org.uk) to get this changed. The development of something like an Institute of Vocational Rehabilitation, as mooted at recent National Employment and Health Innovations Network meetings and the development of standards of practice and competencies to practice may be the start of a newly recognised profession. Only time will tell, but it is recognised by many stakeholders that the safety of the client is paramount and as such, providers should be able to say how they maintain a person's physical, psychological and emotional safety. All too often I have heard and known of horror stories myself where clients have been damaged by their experience of some service providers of vocational rehabilitation.

Does vocational rehabilitation have a role in your workplace?

Do you work with young adults and working aged adults? If the answer is yes, vocational rehabilitation should have a role in your workplace. Does your workplace have the will to include it and develop services to meet clients' needs? That is a totally different question that a book cannot answer. It is not difficult to ask all your clients, patients and service users the 'work' question:

- What about work?
- Are you employed?
- Does your employer know you are off sick and having difficulty coping with work?
- How can I help you make the return to work as easy as possible, perhaps I can call your employer and speak to them?
- What will help you to stay at work and be able to cope?
- What kind of work would you think you are capable of at the moment?
- What kind of career have you been considering?
- What do you think you are good at?
- When do you think you will able to get back to work?
- How will you know when you are ready to work again?
- Tell me about the different working options you have considered?

These questions are not difficult to ask and may in fact prevent someone from needlessly losing their job, falling into financial debt and social exclusion. How work is truly opened up to everyone at all points of service delivery in health, social care and welfare and social exclusion minimised would fill another book and cannot, unfortunately, be addressed competently here.

Your assessments of your clients needs to be well thought out and related to work, using the language of work – not medical language that means nothing except to other similar professionals. Most employers are unlikely to understand medical language, and anyway it is inappropriate. If vocational rehabilitation services are helping people into working, they should be using language that is appropriate. Some of the functional language that is recommended in this book is introduced in Chapter 2 and then continued throughout the rest of the book. Whether someone has a certain strength grading in their quadriceps muscles may be quite important to lower limb range of movement and gait, but this kind of language needs to be translated into non-medical terms such as walking tolerances, or ability to climb stairs.

> Make a list of the terminology you use to describe the function of your clients and then translate this into terms that are related to the functional demands of work.

Assessments are not the entirety of vocational rehabilitation interventions and there needs to be a period of analysis of the assessment information to devise an appropriate plan. Chapter 3 deals with problem solving methods and goal setting with clients. If you do not set goals with your clients, how do you measure their achievements? Service providers need to get into the habit of goal setting as a collaborative process and as required to measure outcomes.

Services have a duty to think of their clients holistically and this includes work whether that is paid or not. However disabled a person seems, they should be offered the chance to achieve the aspirations they believe in. Who are we to doubt that they can achieve great things? This is the time to challenge the service you work in, to plan how to help people achieve occupational mastery and serve occupational justice for everyone.

Summary

In this chapter we have considered vocational rehabilitation in its contemporary context, explaining some of the history associated with what we now see in the UK as vocational rehabilitation. Some of the driving forces of vocational re-habilitation have been considered and the essence of work has also been explored, as well as some of the international contributions and the range of support that may be available. The topic of vocational rehabilitation has been introduced and some challenges have been made to include vocational rehabilitation or at least work in every health and social care service and related services. The future of these service providers is very hard to determine at the moment and it is an excit-ing time to see what develops over the next decade. Will the services start to fit the client any better than they do at the moment? Can creativity be used to design new types of vocational services that do not pigeonhole people into convenient service programmes? Let us all hope that we can add to the body of evidence about vocational rehabilitation by designing our service carefully, thoroughly and capable of producing useful outcomes – as well as striving to do the best by our service users by having them represented on the staff panel and management.

Chapter 2
ASSESSMENT STRATEGIES IN VOCATIONAL REHABILITATION

Introduction

Assessing people for return to work is a broad area, covering many professional and non-professional disciplines and it is not the intention of this text to cover all eventualities. The information in this chapter will relate to those groups of people who are returning to open employment and will aim to address a range of disability and health issues, not focusing on any one in particular. Hagedorn (2000) describes an analytical framework that can be used in the initial stages of contact with a client (Table 2.1). It is, in my opinion, a useful framework for all practitioners because, in a logical sequence of enquiry, it helps us to:

- Organise information gathering
- Assist the practitioner and client to identify problems
- Select priorities and goals

Hagedorn goes on to say that these stages should be used flexibly rather than the rigid stages in which they appear. So, in one session with a client you might go through several stages, or you may have to retrace to a previous stage. It is meant as a guide only, a point of reference to ensure that all the stages of enquiry are considered.

Assessment is not seen as a one-off occasion where strengths and weaknesses are identified, but an ongoing process of discovery about the person you are working with. While initial goals are often necessary to help everybody focus on the ensuing rehabilitation, these are not set in stone and are reactive to the unique circumstances of the individual. When an assessment is carried out, the assessor should be considering the likely outcomes and how the information is to be used effectively and efficiently. There is little reason in carrying out a battery of assessments if the results are never assimilated and acted upon. Assessments are tools and part of a process and a powerful one at that. Even the simple questionnaire should be administered with the thought and awareness that it will be changing people's thoughts, feelings and ultimately their behaviours. *Do be mindful of your own influence over another individual.*

This chapter aims to inform the reader of some ways of organising assessments related to return to work, as well as some of the main areas to consider as part of the assessment process. It is not meant to be a recipe, followed just as it is written. It is anticipated that the reader will use their own professional decision making abilities to choose the right pathway for their client(s).

Table 2.1 The 5 stages of an analytical framework for use in the initial stages of contact.

Stage	Action	Outcome
1. Profiling	Carry out interview and assessments Make initial hypotheses	Written record Baseline data Acceptance by the client of the need for some intervention
2. Naming the problem	Determine what the problems are	Identify a list of problems and some description of the problem(s)
3. Framing the problem	Determine some likely causes and discuss them to facilitate problem solving	Detailed description of the problem(s) recorded in records
4. Prioritise	Explore personal priorities, needs and goals Agree the boundaries of intervention	A record of agreed priorities
5. Action plan	Problem-solving Discussing potential solutions Goal setting Outcome measures Actions to be taken	A record of the goals, outcome measures and action plan

Adapted from Hagedorn (2000), pp. 77–78.

This case study gives you an example of a real situation. Use it to reflect on the issues and comments made in this chapter about assessment. You may want to use a case study of your own to make it more appropriate to your own service or area of expertise.

Case study: John

John works in a local supermarket and he has come to see you because he is having low back pain that is making some of his work tasks impossible to fulfil without making his pain worse. He has had some sharp pain and tingling down one leg for six weeks and has been off work for three weeks now. His job involves moving and lifting boxes around the warehouse and the shop and driving a fork lift for moving pallets. He has a sick note for two more weeks. He is worrying about how he will manage his job and this is affecting his sleep.

Sometimes considering a new way of thinking about service provision can take a while, especially if we are socialised to consider people and situations in a particular way. I am an occupational therapist and as such am socialised into the occupational therapy way of thinking about clients – how have you been socialised and how has your clinical reasoning been affected?

Assessing work function

Work functioning is complex and assessment focuses on the ability of the person to undertake work tasks and to identify the obstacles that are present and preventing them from returning to their chosen work environment. When an individual is not able to work or the capacity to work is reduced, there are social and economic consequences for both the individual and society. Assessment involves understanding that a person's social standing in their community and society in the larger context is often closely associated with their ability to do their work – and assessment of these abilities may alter the perceptions of other people and change relationships. In *Core Curriculum for Professional Education in Pain*, Charlton (2005) states

> 'The decision by a worker to be absent from work is not directly predicted by clinical features or the physical demands of work, but is a complex interaction among occupational, individual and psychosocial factors.'

This statement is taken from research carried out by Dionne (1999), Burton and Main (2000), Waddell et al. (2003).

Assessment can be defined as

> 'The act of assessing . . . evaluation . . . to judge.' (Collins Concise Dictionary 1989)

Assessments can be used to help and advise someone off sick about their return to work. They can help to answer questions such as:

- What should I do to get back to work?
- Will I get back to work?
- Am I suitable for rehabilitation?

Assessments can be designed to contain a *predictive* element – either attempting to predict the type of rehabilitation programme that will assist a return to work; or predicting such things as whether the person is likely to benefit from work rehabilitation or if the person will be able to do their job.

There are many ways to carry out assessments, many types of assessments and a multitude of potential issues to assess as part of someone's returning to the workplace. So what do you look at or investigate? How do you organise or structure your assessments? What types of assessments do you choose? And how do you put them together in a logical framework?

Return to work assessment relating to the person specifically can be seen in three broad areas:

- Work skills
- Work behaviours
- Work tolerance (Northern Ireland Committee of the College of Occupational Therapists 1992)

These three areas pertain to the person, so the other area that requires careful assessment is that of the environment – the workplace and the communities in which the worker travels getting to and from the workplace. Combined with this is the concept that people do not live in a vacuum and that:

'An individual's ability to perform activities is not a static phenomenon.' *(Sandqvist & Henriksson 2004)*

and is influenced by the person themselves, their goals and the circumstances in which the person is carrying out work tasks (Nordenfelt 1996, cited in Sandqvist & Henriksson 2004). So there is a societal context, too. It is not enough to just assess one domain, such as range of movement or intelligence. One needs to evaluate the whole person, their psychological aspirations and the environments in which they work (and get to and from work).

Knowing what to include in an assessment does not necessarily achieve excellence in practice. Looking at how rigorously assessments were carried out, Innes and Straker (2002) suggested that different work-related assessments have different attributes and therefore required different strategies to administer. The results also suggested that to determine high levels of rigour, one might apply guidelines similar to those applied to research methodology. Their advice is that the assessor conducting work-related assessments should:

- Be an experienced professional with appropriate qualifications and training
- Engage in self-reflection
- Obtain impartial feedback through peer review or debriefing

The research recommends that the client should *always* be a main source of data and that data collection should *always* involve interview and observation. The data should be analysed frequently, using a triangulation method. Detailed, structured and coherent reports of the assessments need to be produced, together with audit trails to show how conclusions were established.

Innes and Straker also asked about the barriers in Australia to achieving ideal practice. This was reported as the time available and costs of equipment/assessment systems, and the unwillingness of parties to pay for detailed reports. While acknowledging that there is an ideal to strive for, the actual assessment processes need to be realistic, workable and appropriate for the individual set of circumstances. If you are lucky enough to work in a situation where you have control over what you do and spend, then you might be able to achieve the utmost and assess everyone in his or her own work environment. However, if you are a junior member of staff and work in the acute sector of the healthcare system with little time on your hands and no specialist equipment, you will need to adjust what you are feasibly able to carry out. You may find that you are only able to manage some of the person-based and very few of the environment-based assessments, and none of the function-based assessments. Whatever your situation, you can always look to evidence your practices, use the assessment information wisely and continuously push for better and more appropriate services for your clients.

The assessment aims to:

- Identify the barriers (obstacles) that prevent the person coming off sick leave and returning to their own workplace
- Provide data that can be analysed to categorise barriers and determine the interrelationships
- Provide information to establish the appropriate interventions to assist with a return to work

What might be the aims of assessment for John?

What are the aims of assessment for your service?

To simplify the huge topic of assessment and the array of possible protocols, types and equipment available, the following sections will cover most of the pertinent areas mentioned above. The categorising is somewhat artificial because in reality you may well be addressing several issues from these three main categories simultaneously. They are separated here to provide some organised structure and a checklist.

Person-based assessments address those issues pertaining to the whole person and include looking at physical assessments, yellow flags, blue flags, work behaviours and work skills.

Environment-based assessments address issues pertaining to the environment, including the community, and include topics on black flags, work site assessment, job analysis and work relationships.

Function-based assessments address those issues around the person carrying out the work task and address work tolerance, job matching and functional capacity evaluations.

To manage the assessment process you may find it helpful to think about it in stages, asking yourself various questions as you go along (Figure 2.1).

Core assessment

As in most services when a new referral is received, basic information is collected first – so it is in return to work programmes. This first encounter with your client might be called a core assessment, as it contains the core information required before further detailed assessments are recommended. The assessment would usually be conducted face-to-face with your client, in a private room to maintain confidentiality and with some basic comforts such as appropriate seating and tables, water to drink, tissues, and a 'do not disturb' sign on the door. The first session can be a release for your client as they tell you about their unique story – so you need to be ready for a whole range of emotions to be expressed. This first encounter may take anywhere between 45 minutes and two hours to conduct.

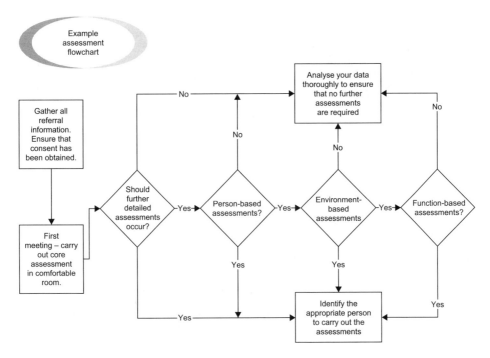

Figure 2.1 Example assessment flowchart.

Table 2.2 is a list of basic information that you may be able to obtain from your client in an interview and also from reading prior reports and records if this is appropriate in your service.

You may want to devise a form that allows you to write down some or all of the information as your client tells it to you during the core assessment. However,

Table 2.2 Basic assessment information.

Demographics This information would usually come as part of the referral process	Names Age (date of birth) Address Telephone numbers (home, mobile, workplace(s), next of kin)
Medical history This will generally only come from the client, unless you have consent to see medical record or talk with medical professionals	GP name and contact details Reason for sick leave Details of sick notes (duration of current one especially) Previous occurrences of the same issues Family history of the same or related issues Other people in the workplace with similar condition (not names, just numbers) Known risk factors or related conditions Investigations carried out Treatment received/referred and waiting for Health insurance Contributory health schemes

Table 2.2 *continued.*

Social situation It is important to ascertain the client's circumstances as this can affect certain issues	House type (owner occupied, council owned, privately rented) House style (bungalow, semi-detached, flat etc.) Living arrangements (alone, with partner, with other relatives, friends etc.) Dependants
Social support Covers the immediate family and the larger community	Emotional support Physical support Financial support Car driver Community transport
Financial information Important information can be gathered that can be used to assess the likelihood of your client being able to obtain financial support	Occupational sickness benefit and pay State benefits Savings (certain thresholds will determine certain state benefits) Pay from other jobs (some people do not take sick leave from all their jobs at the same time as only one job may be causing difficulties) Insurance claims (mortgage repayment, other repayment schemes, litigation claims (accidents), income protection schemes)
Current work details Essential to establish if your client is employed or self-employed. Most clients will not know all this information and they may have to go away and find it out	Name of employer, line manager Type and sector of business i.e. transport, large goods transport Address of employer and place of actual work as these can be different Telephone numbers Email addresses, website address Union rep Health and safety rep Human resources contact Occupational health contact Works doctor
Educational background and work history This will give you an idea of the person's career path to date and it will give you an opportunity to enquire about the choices that have been taken	Primary schooling Secondary schooling – left school at what age? Further education – qualifications Literacy Numeracy Dyslexia issues Chronological work history
Daily activities performance There are many ways of assessing these areas; some are based on observations and others on self-reporting questionnaires or interview	Daily living (personal care, dressing, communication, functional mobility, cooking, home management tasks, carer roles) Leisure (existing, previous, desired activities) Educational (formal and informal types)

Table 2.3 Example of an initial action plan following a core assessment.

Issues	Actions	Timeframe
Need more information about John's current investigations with the medical team	John will give written permission to liaise with his consultant and physiotherapist	In 1 week
	Caseworker will talk to the medical practitioners about contraindications related to work tasks	In 2 weeks
Psychological issues related to John's workplace accident	Caseworker will refer John for specialist assessments	3 days
	John will be seen by the cognitive behavioural psychotherapist	In 1 month
John needs to know basic information about his rights as an employee off sick from work	Caseworker will mail John some relevant information	1 week
	The caseworker will call John regularly	Every 2 weeks
	John will return after his specialist assessment to look at his rehabilitation plan	5 weeks

remember that writing and listening are not easy tasks to do simultaneously – and do ask your client's permission to write down what they tell you. Try not to solve all the issues in this first meeting. Ask your client to tell you his or her story, listen to your client, and understand what they are feeling and the events that have led them to see you. Be very careful not to make judgements or assumptions on the minimal information you will have gathered at this stage. Instead, attempt to develop a clear picture of who they are as an individual and the personal journey that has brought them to see you.

At the end of this first interview, you and your client can decide what the next steps should be. You might find it handy to write these decisions down so that you both go away with exactly the same information (Table 2.3).

It is your responsibility to make it clear:

- What the next steps will be
- Who will contact your client (you, an administrator, another colleague)
- How they will be contacted (telephone, email, letter)
- When they should expect to be contacted – if your service cannot see them for three months, tell your client this, don't say that you will speak to them 'soon'

Table 2.4 Clinical reasoning in SOAP notes.

S(ubjective)	John reports that he feels nervous about returning to work with the pain he is experiencing. He is unsure about going into work for an assessment
O(bjective)	John became sweaty when discussing work, thoughts became somewhat rushed and not thought through
A(nalysis)	Workplace-based assessments should be held off until the psychological elements are addressed
	Keep discussing the workplace throughout assessments
P(lan)	Give John confidence by allowing him time to get accustomed to his pain and maintaining activity levels
	Give John relevant information regarding pain John will consider consent for further psychological assessments with cognitive behavioural therapist

What next?

Once the core assessment has been carried out, you may have the skills, time and resources to start looking at more of the specific issues that your client has raised. You may need to carry out some person-based assessments, some environment-based assessments and some function-based assessments. Choosing what is appropriate to do next is important and should be considered carefully. It may not be appropriate to do function-based assessments before analysing what the job entails by looking at the work environment. Likewise, it may not be safe to take your client to the workplace to do an environment-based assessment if you have not checked out his or her pain or anxiety, i.e. person-based assessment.

Consider how you will provide a trail to show your decision making and how your assessment process is designed to be rigorous. For instance, in your clinical notes you could document clearly the reasons behind designing the assessments in the way you do. An example can be seen in Table 2.4. You may not use SOAP notes yourself (Subjective–Objective–Analysis–Plan) but you may able to see how the clinical reasoning can be documented in an ordinary set of notes.

Person-based assessments

Here we look at some of the person-based assessment areas that are usually targeted when looking at someone who is off sick from work. Once you have completed the core assessment you will need to make some initial decisions about the detailed assessments that are required.

Have you identified issues that will require a physical examination such as pain, mobility problems, balance difficulties, headaches, pins and needles, fatigue and so on?

Have you identified issues that will require further psychological investigations such as low mood, anxieties, fear, poor coping strategies and so on?

Have you identified issues that will require further cognitive assessment such as memory loss, difficulties with concentration or poor problem solving abilities?

Let us look at some more specific assessments that target issues for those people who are off sick from work. As mentioned previously, the three broad areas related to assessment can be described as: work skills, work behaviours and work tolerance. We will cover these areas but focus on the categories of physical assessments, psychological assessments, work behaviours and skills. As mentioned already, the division of the following areas is academic because in practice you will be assessing several areas simultaneously, especially as you become more experienced.

Assessing physical functioning

The purpose of assessing physical functioning is to provide a functional baseline of the neuromusculoskeletal system so that changes in function can be measured as the client works towards their safe functional limitations (Matheson 2004). A physical functioning assessment would normally identify those problems that are contributing to your client's obstacles in returning to work and cover previous relevant history, past medical history and present injury or illness.

Specifically, one could use assessments to:

- Identify or exclude clinical red flags indicating serious pathology requiring secondary care.
- Identify specific pathology and/or dysfunctions in particular joints and tissues such as muscle weakness, restricted range of movement, poor postural control. This should lead to a diagnosis or a hypothesis about why the injury has occurred and from which a prognosis can be sought and treatment plan created.
- Identify the impact of the specific dysfunction for home and work activities such as sitting and walking.
- Focus on posture and alignment, flexibility and mobility, strength, neurological examination and gait.
- Assess specific elements such as:
  - Vertebral artery test: designed to test for compression in the vertebral artery.
  - Quadrant test: designed to test cervical nerve root compression.
  - Tinel's sign: designed to determine carpal tunnel syndrome.

There are many more tests than these, but you need to ask yourself whether you are the right person to conduct these tests and the physical functioning assessment per se. Physiotherapists have physical functioning as a core part of their training and are therefore experienced in this area of assessment. As Innes and Straker (2002) suggested, part of the rigour of assessments is to ensure that the assessor is suitably qualified.

Physical job demands

Innes (1997) in Pratt and Jacobs (1997) suggests that the neuromusculoskeletal and motor components most commonly affected in work-related problems are those of

'strength, range of movement, endurance (both cardiorespiratory and muscle endurance), postural alignment and fine coordination/dexterity.'

It is important at this stage to talk a little of physical job demands (Table 2.5).

Job demands are those physical demands that each work task makes on the person carrying them out. So, some jobs can involve lifting and carrying but not stair or ladder work, for instance a warehouse worker. Some jobs will involve fine finger dexterity, light and firm grasp, forward sitting and visual perception, for instance a lab technician. You should be able to have the job demands of your client's work listed or at least in your mind when you are carrying out physical functioning assessments to ensure that you are targeting your assessments appropriately.

Table 2.5 Summary of physical job demands.

Component	Job demand	Component	Job demand
Strength	Lifting	**Dexterity**	Fine finger
	Carrying		Grasp – light
	Pushing		Grasp – firm
	Pulling		Pinching
Mobility	Sitting		Writing
	Dynamic standing		Handling
	Static standing		Reaching upwards
	Walking		Reaching forwards
Agility	Stairs/ladders		Foot controls
	Balancing	**Co-ordination**	Eye-hand
	Crouching/kneeling		Eye-hand-foot
	Stooping	**Vision/hearing**	Visual perception
	Bending		Near acuity (< 20 inches)
	Twisting/spinal rotation		Far acuity (> 20 feet)
	Above shoulder work		Colour vision
	Low level work		Depth perception
			Hearing

You might be intrigued about someone's visual perception abilities, but if it is not a demand of their job is it valid to make an assessment of that area?

You will need to choose an appropriate environment in which to carry out your physical functioning examination. You may need to have your client partially undressed to carry out some assessments and so privacy and an area to undress and dress will be required. You will need appropriate equipment, at the very least a chair and floor area and you may find a goniometer, dynamometer, tape measure and a treatment couch useful, too. With the correct consent forms signed, you may want to video or take photos of your client carrying out movements so that you can analyse them carefully later on. You will need to decide whether you should do the assessment alone, or if assistance may be required, e.g. some balance testing is safer carried out with more than one person in case the person starts to fall.

It is not appropriate to explain a full musculoskeletal examination in this text. If you need to learn how to do this, I would encourage you to search out the appropriate professional development in the form of a course, or tutoring from a physiotherapist, for instance. Remember this learning will be part of your continuing professional development, so document it in a relevant way so you have your evidence to show if required.

You may have developed specialised skills to assess physical functioning – if so, you will know what assessments to carry out and how to carry them out. However, for those who are not specialists, there are some basic areas at which you may want to look. Ruling out serious pathology using red flags has already been mentioned and is important to establish whether there is indication for further medical/surgical investigations therefore lessening the risk of secondary damage.

Remembering John's case study (p. 19), John is in pain and has some tingling and shooting sensations down his leg. It seems reasonable first to rule out any serious pathology. Initial discussion would include looking at the presenting problem(s). In John's case that would be establishing how long the symptoms had been bothering him, and if there was a definite event that caused the pain to start.

It is important to gauge the client's perception of those problems early on as this starts to tell you how much of an issue the symptoms are. In John's case you would ask about his pain (symptom) history, which would also include the site of the pain, severity of the pain, behaviour associated with the pain including fear–avoidance behaviours. Some people start to avoid certain activities because the pain worsens and sometimes there can be associated thoughts or beliefs that the pain is informing them to stop because more damage will occur if they carry on with the activity. John needs to understand his pain and not assume that pain means he has to stop all activities that exacerbate his symptoms. As John has been presented to you early on in his sick leave, you may have a good opportunity to either prevent or stop these thoughts and beliefs before they become ingrained.

Pain questionnaires and scales

You may want to use some pain questionnaires or pain scales to help to understand your client's symptoms. Some examples are shown in Box 2.1.

Box 2.1　Pain questionnaires and scales.

Matheson Functional Pain Scale (Matheson 2002): See Table 2.6.

Oswestry Low Back Disability Questionnaire (Fairbank et al. 1980): A 10 item, self-report questionnaire shown to be valid in looking at perceived disability. It is quick to administer and relevant to everyday life situations.

Neck Disability Index (NDI) (Vernon and Mior 1991): Developed from the Oswestry Low Back Pain Questionnaire and is similar in its administration and relevance to daily life.

McGill Pain Questionnaire (Melzack 1975): Relevant for any pain, and not just back pain. It is designed to look at the multidimensional nature of the pain experience (Turk & Melzack 1992). There are 20 groups of words used to describe pain and the client is asked to work through each group identifying a word in each that represents their symptoms.

Dallas Pain Questionnaire (DPQ) (Lawlis et al. 1989): Looks at chronic spinal pain and uses similar dimensions as the Oswestry questionnaires. It therefore has relevance to everyday situations and it has factors that address work. Its interpretation is said to be able to determine the most appropriate type of treatment i.e. medical treatment only, combination of medical and behavioural interventions.

Some questionnaires can also be used as outcome measures and you may find that this is useful for your service area. However, as with all tools, you should think carefully which one will answer the questions you have about your client and the questions your client has about him or herself. Standardised tools are useful and have their place in assessment, but using them for the sake of ease or apparent evidence base may not reflect the individual needs of your client or service.

An important reason for having pain questionnaires is to gain an understanding of:

- What your client does to cope with their pain
- What thoughts they have about their pain
- How much this coping behaviour helps or hinders their return to work

Details of medication might have been established in the core assessment, but in my experience not everyone has this information to hand unless you can see the person in their own home. It is important to be aware of the types of medication someone takes – and its effect and possible side effects. But even if you are not an expert in the types of medication, it would seem sensible to know what the medication is called, when they take it, how long they have been taking it and whether they manage to stick to the dose that has been prescribed or advised.

Table 2.6 Matheson Functional Pain Scale.

Functional Pain Scale			
Please choose a description that best describes the functional effect of your pain. Feel free to use half points if the effect of your pain is somewhat higher or somewhat lower than any specific description.			
10		Immediate emergency hospitalisation	Worst pain imaginable. Requires **immediate emergency hospitalisation**. Causes you to be completely incapacitated and barely able to talk.
9			Pain that causes disability between levels 7 and 10. Nearing need for hospitalisation.
8			
7		Severely disabling pain	**Severely disabling pain**. You cannot use or move the painful area. You have difficulty speaking and/or engaging in conversation. You have difficulty concentrating on anything but the pain. **Needing to lie down and pain-related tearfulness** are also common at this level of pain.
6			Pain that causes disability between levels 5 and 7.
5		Very disabling pain	**Very disabling pain**. Causes great difficulty moving or applying any strength through the painful area. You would **stop using the painful area** for the present activity.
4			Pain that causes disability between levels 3 and 5.
3		Visibly disabling pain	Pain is starting to **visibly disable** you. It is starting to cause difficulty moving or applying strength through the painful area, affecting your productivity or performance. Causes you to take small breaks to rest or stretch.
2			**Non-disabling pain** or discomfort. Does not impair ability to move fully, with normal speed or strength.
1			
0.5		Non-disabling pain	
0		No pain	**No pain** or discomfort.

(Reproduced with permission from Roy Matheson, The Matheson System)

If John (case study p. 19) has had days when he has had to resort to extra medication, this might be a clue as to the severity of his pain and his coping strategies.

Musculoskeletal examination would include range of movement (active and passive movements) and functional muscle strength. John has explained that he cannot lift and move the boxes at work any more so it will be important to understand if he has associated reductions in movement and strength.

Specific tests can be employed to look at these areas, such as repeated range of movement tests, for example bending to reach the floor (stooping). The test involves a full range of movement tests first, followed by 10 repetitions of the same movement at a pace comfortable to the client and then 10 repetitions as fast as is possible, recording the time and the behaviours exhibited during the test. As far as is known, there are no normative data with which to compare your client, and the behavioural observations and client feedback are more likely to be of value. These examinations will tell you how he or she functions now – but they will not tell you how he or she needs to be or how he or she is able to function at work until you carry out more function-based assessments and environment, i.e. worksite assessments.

John's posture is likely to be changed as he holds himself differently to help to minimise his pain. Further aches and pains can start because of this behaviour and this may complicate the picture. John's postural stability around his trunk may be compromised because his deep stabilising muscles are firing slowly and this will not assist him to support his back or maintain a correct posture/alignment while working (Box 2.2). He is also experiencing some associated altered proprioception as well as altered sensation in one leg and so his gait and movements may be affected overall. He might be quite stiff when he walks, which may have an impact on how quickly he can move and agile he is. In his line of work he needs to be able to move quickly and effectively, as he has to shift a certain number of boxes in a day.

Box 2.2 Postural stability.

The deep stabilising muscles in the trunk play a role in maintaining posture and alignment during functional activity. The muscles become inhibited by pain – their timing delayed and so they do not respond quickly enough during activity and leave the body vulnerable to further injury or strain. This is called functional instability by physiotherapists – where a person may be able to hold a posture in a test but fails in everyday activities that are repeated normally because the muscles are firing too slowly. They are slow rather than weak.

Treatment is aimed at restoring the timing and integrating the muscle activation into function. If stability is not restored even after the pain has resolved, the person may be open to recurrent episodes of similar types of problems.

Other useful information can be gained from questionnaires that focus on how the client sees themselves and their symptoms. One such questionnaire is the Disabilities of the Arm, Shoulder and Hand (DASH) Outcome Measure. It is

'A 30-item, self-report questionnaire designed to measure physical function and symptoms in patients with any or several musculoskeletal disorders of the upper limb. The questionnaire was designed to help describe the disability experienced by people with upper-limb disorders and also to monitor changes in symptoms and function over time.' (Institute for Work and Health and the American Academy of Orthopaedic Surgeons)

Videoing clients moving around is a recognised part of assessment for many physiotherapists and if you have consent to do this, it allows you more time to look in depth and repeatedly at behaviour and movement patterns.

If you are able to video John at work on a trial, even better. A close second might be videoing someone else doing his job. This would give you a comparison between John's actual ability to bend, reach, stoop etc and how other people perform these actions in the workplace.

Summary

In a physical functioning assessment you would normally expect to help to identify those problems that are contributing to your client's obstacles in returning to work. It may cover previous relevant history, past medical history, present injury or illness, posture and alignment, flexibility and mobility, strength, neurological examination, gait and special tests in relation to the job demands of your client's workplace.

Psychological and behavioural assessments

The purpose of broad psychological assessments is to provide a functional baseline of mood, cognition and memory so that changes in function can be assessed as the client moves towards greater occupational independence. Assessments will normally cover the relevant history of current symptoms and issues. The assessments themselves will most heavily rely on the narrative your client will tell you about him or herself. They may also include psychometric testing, psychometric questionnaires (personality trait types for instance), neuropsychological tests, standardised questionnaires (looking at anxiety for instance) and observations of behaviour. The goal is to investigate how these issues might affect working abilities and competency with the aim of identifying what functional support is required in the work place as well as remediating symptoms to enable your client to successfully carry out their work tasks.

When referring to individuals with severe cognitive disorders and to standard psychological assessments, McCue et al. (1994) explain that:

'These assessments provided information on intellectual capacity and academic achievement but often failed to address the issues of reasonable vocational goals, possible obstacles and rehabilitation strategies.'

They go on to imply that these issues could be improved by integrating information to do with worksite demands into the interpretation of the results.

Cognition per se is usually assessed separately to mental health issues. If you are already experienced in these areas, you will be able to choose from a range of tools with which you are already familiar.

Value in the workplace

Donaldson (1997) in Pratt and Jacobs (1997) talks about how businesses recognise value in the workplace. He explains that value is perceived in economic terms:

'The source of value can be directly from the performance of an employee.'

Donaldson goes on to describe value in terms of tangible elements such as the actual work completed and intangible value elements including

'morale, team spirit, co-operation, dependability, reliability and consistency.'

With regard to the work environment, one would be considering broad psychological functions such as memory, productivity, safety and interpersonal behaviour, sometimes known as feasibility. This is defined by Leonard Matheson as

'the acceptability of the worker in the general sense i.e., worker traits and behaviours.' (Matheson 2004)

James Japp (2005), describing cognitive assessments for brain injury, also describes a similar list that he calls executive skills. Table 2.7 shows the accepted (North American) list of psychosocial types of job demands:

The whole picture

Table 2.7 is useful in structuring the overall assessment process, but it is based on functional capacity evaluation, where there is a heavy focus on physical function and not psychological functioning. In simplifying things we are at risk of missing vital areas to address. Another note of caution when considering assessment for return to work is the appropriateness of assessing every deficit you might uncover. If your primary role is to look at return to work, then you should be aware of the psychological job demands of your client's job before you start addressing every issue that is raised. For instance, is it relevant for you to address past traumatic events as part of a return to work programme? Someone may need to address them, but is it you? Likewise, if someone is self-employed, works at home but has anxiety about leaving the house, should you address this problem as part of a return to work programme?

Table 2.7 Psychosocial types of job demands.

Component	Job demand	Component	Job demand
Cognition	Understanding instructions Memory Concentration/attention	Safety	Adherence to safety rules Use of proper body mechanics Use of protective behaviour
Productivity	Quantity Quality Attendance Timeliness	Interpersonal behaviour	Response to supervision Response to co-workers Response to change Attitude to work/role

Adapted from Roy Matheson Associates Inc, course notes relating to the Matheson System of functional capacity evaluations (2004) with permission from Roy Matheson, The Matheson System.

McCue et al. (1994) explain that one of the main difficulties with individuals with cognitive disabilities is realistic self-appraisal. They suggest that a positive outcome from assessments is an agreement between the client and the other people involved in the assessment process, regarding their current return to work obstacles and strategies that might help to overcome these. There needs to be less emphasis on the impairment and more focus on framing problems in real life and vocationally relevant issues, for example:

'I have a memory problem' might be rephrased as 'I find it difficult to take telephone messages and pass them on accurately.'

From a business perspective, these more intangible factors are said to influence the perception of value in the workplace and Donaldson (in Pratt & Jacobs 1997) proposes that:

'To obtain and maintain employment, a person needs to be perceived as contributing "value", as understood by the particular organisation.'

Leach (2002) also describes a similar range that employers are looking for in their employees. These subtle skills in the most part make up workplace competency, which again need to be viewed on an individual basis for each employer. This then will give a sense of what is deemed as valuable. If you know what is seen as valuable in an organisation, you then have another factor to which you can match your client's abilities. It also helps to identify where there might be a mismatch – this information helps you to design intervention for a return to work programme.

Work behaviours

Human resource personnel are used to looking at workplace competency and recognise how this relates to value in an organisation. Charles Woodruffe (1992), a human resource expert, says that competency in the workplace is *'the set of behaviour patterns that the incumbent needs to bring to a position to perform its tasks and functions.'*

This idea is widely used in workplaces in Britain already. One of the ways of looking at psychological aspects will be to observe behaviours that are exhibited, preferably in the workplace or in a situation similar to the workplace. Is your client demonstrating appropriate responses to a supervisor, or co-workers? Does your client turn up to appointments on time? How does your client respond to changes?

Work behaviours can also be defined as

'the conduct of a person in the work situation.' (Northern Ireland Committee of College of Occupational Therapists 1992)

This group also subdivided work behaviours into work attitudes, work habits and work traits (Table 2.8).

Some of these aspects can be observed, such as punctuality, initiative and interpersonal skills; while some are part of the belief system of an individual, such as work values, self-confidence and self-motivation. Observation of such elements is not possible and different methods are needed, such as questionnaires or a narrative approach. Checklists or structured interview are useful tools to guide the assessor. An example of this would be the Worker Role Interview (Velozo et al. 1998), which is elaborated on later in this chapter. Another similar style used in supported employment is the vocational profile (Leach 2002). Both attempt to tease out the strengths that a person has in relation to what is required in a workplace and workplace competency.

You will be able to identify many more areas to assess in relation to your client if your expertise is in this domain. The responsible practitioner recognises when it is necessary to refer on to a more qualified specialist.

Table 2.8 Categories of work behaviours.

Work attitudes	Work habits	Work traits
The expression of the person's thoughts and feelings towards his or her work	The regular tendencies of the person	The characteristics of the person
Work values, work motivation, work ambitions, worker role, and attitude to authority	Attendance, punctuality, safety consciousness, accuracy, concentration	Reliability, responsibility, self-confidence, adaptability, initiative, speed, perseverance

Northern Ireland Committee of College of Occupational Therapists, 1992

If in our case study John (p. 19) had a history of complex psychological issues or enduring mental health problems you might want to explore how these affect his ability to work and meet his job demands competently. You might do this in conjunction with a mental health worker, a health psychologist or a cognitive behavioural psychotherapist to name but a few relevant professionals. Obviously, your choice is dependent on your service's restrictions, the availability of the professional as well as the costs of the individual specialist.

There are a wide range of tests that help clinically when addressing cognitive, mental health and psychological issues/problems, too many to possibly name in this book. Again you need to ask yourself whether you are the right person to carry out and interpret these assessments and how relevant or useful they are in the process of helping someone to return to work. Many of these tests measure discrete functions or symptoms that are not directly transferable to a workplace. It is necessary, therefore to apply the results of the tests to the work environment, which leaves much to one's personal interpretation and possible mistakes.

As with the core assessment, where you choose to carry out these psychological-based assessments should be considered. While the assessment will be mostly narrative, i.e. talking, you may still need to consider the basics such as tissues, and water to drink. You should also be aware of the soundproofing in the assessment environment. Let your client know if it is not soundproof, so that they can moderate the volume of their conversation adequately.

Independent of the primary cause for sickness absence, psychological factors are seen as having an immense effect on return to work. Psychological factors are important areas to address in musculoskeletal symptoms as well as those symptoms associated more commonly with brain injury or mental health.

Yellow Flags

Some fundamental aspects of assessment in return to work were developed in response to the vast numbers of people being off sick from work because of back pain in the latter part of the 20th century. In 1997 three clinical psychologists, Kendall, Linton and Main developed the concept of 'Yellow Flags' – psychological risk factors that identify those people at risk of developing chronic disability. Yellow Flags have had an international impact on all consequent guidelines associated with back pain and now are used in relation to a wider range of pain-related conditions (Working Backs Scotland, www.workingbacksscotland.com). There is a growing body of evidence to suggest that a person's belief about himself or herself has a profound effect on whether a return to work will be successful. Charlton (2005) uses the research of several authors (Burton & Main 2000, Main & Burton 2000, Waddell & Burton 2000) to state:

'Psychosocial factors are the main determinants of disability and are significant predictors of prolonged work absence in painful conditions.'

Table 2.9 Risk factors 'flags'.

Flags	Purpose	Developed by
Red	Identify physical risk factors and the development of serious disease	Agency for Health Care Policy and Research (AHCPR) 1994
	Involves a thorough physical examination by a physician or physiotherapist who can identify the need for further investigations and possible surgical intervention	
	Includes features of neurological disease, significant trauma, weight loss, history of cancer, fever, intravenous drug use, steroid use, people over 50 years old, severe night time pain, pain worsening when lying down	
Yellow	Identify psychological risk factors and development of chronic disability using a questionnaire	Kendall et al. 1997
	Include distress, depression, coping strategies, disadvantageous beliefs	
Orange	Identify psychiatric risks and development of psychological and psychiatric illness	Main et al. 2005 cited in Reidy-Crofts (online)
	Used to identify when a psychiatric opinion should be sought	
Blue	Identify perceptions of the worker and will differ from person to person in the same workplace. Look at worker-specific personal factors such as blame, beliefs about the work/injury relationship, perceived work demands, psychosocial aspects of work	Main & Burton 2000
Black	Identify factors external to the person including the occupational environment and reflect the employer's perceptions and attitudes	Main & Burton 1998, 2000; Waddell & Burton 2004
	Include organisational policies, processes and practices about return to work and rehabilitation	

There are other coloured flags to assist with assessment (Table 2.9).

The evidence around one's beliefs has already been mentioned in the context of the Yellow Flags and back pain. The evidence available surrounding individuals' beliefs about return to work are compelling reading in the subject areas of career decision making, musculoskeletal problems and psychological issues. The need to address your client's beliefs about return to work is part of their overall assessment.

Self-efficacy
Albert Bandura (1995) coined and then developed the term self-efficacy, which he defines as a

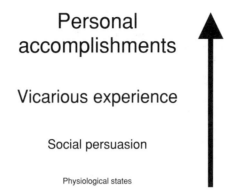

Personal accomplishments

Vicarious experience

Social persuasion

Physiological states

Figure 2.2 Sources of efficacy expectations.
After Albert Bandura.

'context-specific assessment of competence to perform a specific task or a range of tasks in a given domain – an individual's judgement of his or her capabilities to perform given actions.'

Bandura explains that self-efficacy has the effect of influencing one's choices, effort, how long one persists when faced with obstacles and how one feels. Self-efficacy is said to come from four major sources (Figure 2.2).

You can see from Figure 2.2 that personal accomplishment and mastery is the strongest source of efficacy expectation, and physiological states is the weaker source. What is particularly useful about this model is the practical application it has for people wanting to return to work. In your interview assessment you can ask direct questions about the self-efficacy your client has with regard to the tasks they need to perform at work. Bandura (1995) says:

'A self-efficacy assessment, therefore, includes both an affirmation of a capability level and the strength of that belief.'

So in our case study, John (p. 19) would benefit from being questioned about his self-efficacy in the tasks he has to do in the supermarket to determine how much effort and persistence he might show in the face of the obstacles that may come his way while he considers his pathways to return to work.

There are self-efficacy scales available, but as this concept is context-specific, it is likely to be difficult to find one that will fit your clients' situations all the time. It seems that practitioners need to make good use of their interviewing skills, using the narrative from their clients to gain some understanding of individuals' self-efficacy.

If we help John to become more self-aware, perhaps he is more likely to understand why he feels able to be persistent and give effort in some parts of his return to work programme and not others.

Model of Human Occupation

Another way of considering this part of a psychological-based assessment is founded in occupational therapy theory. One particular theory, the Model of Human Occupation (MOHO) by Gary Kielhofner (1985) has evolved the tools for work assessments. Velozo et al. (1998) use the term personal causation in the work context to mean

'a collection of beliefs and expectations that a person holds about his/her effectiveness in the work environment.'

This is similar to Bandura's concept of self-efficacy. The Worker Role Interview (WRI) is an assessment tool based on MOHO that addresses personal causation and a range of other factors around psychosocial and environmental variables and it looks at the potential a person has to return to work (Velozo et al. 1998). As with many other assessment tools, it is recommended that training is undertaken to administer the tool appropriately. For this tool, if you do not have an occupational therapy background you will benefit from having an understanding of MOHO to fully assimilate the concepts of the WRI or its companion the Work Environment Impact Scale (Moore-Corner et al. 1998).

Summary

In summary, you would normally expect a psychological and behavioural-based assessment to help identify those problems that are contributing to your client's obstacles in return to work. The assessment will also highlight those strengths that your client will rely on to help them in their return to work. It may cover previous relevant history, past medical history, present issues or illness, beliefs, self-efficacy, cognition, productivity, safety and interpersonal behaviour in relation to the job demands of your client's workplace and the workplace competency as perceived by the employer.

Function-based assessments

The purpose of function-based assessments is to provide a baseline of abilities in actual tasks. These might occur in the workplace as real job tasks or in a rehabilitation setting as simulated job tasks making them as real as possible. Function-based assessments combine the physical, psychological and behavioural aspects with the environmental aspects already discussed. McCue (1993) cited in McCue et al. (1994) says:

'Functional assessments go beyond standard approaches . . . and identify functional obstacles to goal attainment, residual job skills, and the specific conditions under which these skills can be utilized.'

Assessments will be guided by the actual or potential job tasks that your client will be doing at work and the environment in which they will be carrying them out. You will be using the information already gathered in previous assessments to design the most appropriate functional assessment and this will give you the chance to see how your client performs. The assessments will rely heavily on observations and you may want to obtain consent to video the session(s) with your client. The goal is to see how close the match is between the job demands and work environment and your client's ability to complete the job tasks, sometimes known as the functional capacity of the client. The assessments should identify any mismatches between these elements and help to guide appropriate interventions and match a person with their appropriate work.

As has already been said:

'An individual's ability to perform activities is not a static phenomenon.'
(Sandqvist & Henriksson 2004)

Nordenfelt 1996 (cited in Sandqvist & Henriksson 2004) proposes three interdependent factors that can hinder or assist an individual to perform work activities:

- The agent (individual) involved
- The goal of this agent
- The circumstances in which the agent acts

Assessment of your client's functional ability to carry out his or her work tasks is a dynamic relationship between the environment, him or herself as an individual and the goals.

A key point here is that the functional assessment is designed to look solely at the job your client has or wants to do – not a wide range of tasks. So where you choose to observe your client is also an important issue to work out before designing the assessment. There is a movement towards assessments being carried out in the workplace because they have more meaning (face validity) and are more realistic (Stuckey 1997; Gibson & Strong 2003; Sandqvist & Henriksson 2004). However, there can be tension between the client and various people in the workplace that might make this setting unfeasible; and there may be health and safety issues that would make it difficult to use the workplace as an assessment environment. Often a strong rapport with the employer helps to make the workplace a more feasible environment in which to make an assessment, but there will still be elements in that environment over which you will have little control. Only you and your client will be able to decide which is the most appropriate place.

Job retention

In this chapter we focus on functional capacity evaluations, job simulation and job matching. But first I wanted to introduce the idea that one can start to identify people who might be struggling at work and to help with job retention, before they have to take time off from work. This obviously has to happen in the workplace itself and might be as part of an occupational health service or a human resources policy on absence management or policies on the welfare of the workers. Alternatively, it could occur in the primary health sector, i.e. when someone visits their general practitioner. There is an inherent difficulty around gathering this information in a workplace because disclosing one's own productivity difficulties at work could be seen as unfavourable to one's position (depending on the attitudes and culture of the organisation). Another difficulty is that one's ability to do the job may be compromised in such a slow and insidious way that it is actually challenging for the person to identify if they are struggling until the situation is almost at crisis point. When a person first develops difficulties at work, such as fatigue, acute pain, headaches or lowered concentration, an employer may have policies to instigate procedures to look at problem solving and so prevent the person from being absent from work or losing their job. The workplace or health professionals may have their own screening tools to assess the likelihood that someone may be struggling and may have to take sick leave. Examples of published screening tools are the Work Instability Scale and the Work Ability Index.

Work Instability Scale

Work instability has been defined as:

> 'A state in which the consequences of a mis-match between an individual's functional (and cognitive) abilities and the demands of their job can threaten continuing employment if not resolved.' (Gilworth et al. 2003)

The Work Instability Scale was developed by the Academic Unit of Musculoskeletal and Rehabilitation Medicine, University of Leeds. It was originally based on back pain and then extended to be relevant for arthritis, traumatic brain injury, multiple sclerosis and epilepsy. It has now been translated into other European languages. Scores on the Work Instability Scale indicate the level of work disability (premature work cessation) and possible need for job retention measures:

0–9   low risk of work disability
10–16   medium risk of work disability
17+   high risk of work disability

The Work Ability Index

The Workplace and Health Information Gateway says that the Work Ability Index

> 'enables workers to signal that they think that they may have problems in the future, and it gives occupational health professionals and managers the opportunity to intervene early to prevent loss of staff.'

The Finnish Institute of Occupational Health originally developed the Work Ability Index in 1981 as a diagnostic tool to support the worker. The tool is said to predict the threat of disability in the near future. It is a questionnaire that can be used for any worker and gives a score that can be interpreted thus:

7–27   poor   restore work ability
28–36   moderate   improve work ability
37–43   good   support work ability
44–49   excellent   maintain work ability

Functional capacity evaluation

Functional capacity evaluations (FCE) have been used in North America since the early to mid 1980s when the term was established. This happened at a time when the occupational rehabilitation industry was growing fast. The importance of FCEs has grown – especially in the USA – as the demand for valid data about the need to identify injured workers' safe return to work (RTW) capacity increases. Clinicians working with clients who are injured and off sick can use the FCE as one of a number of assessments to determine the client's ability to return to work safely *and* at what level of work they should return. It reflects what the client's abilities are at the time of the assessment. In the UK, while there is knowledge of FCEs, the market for this type of assessment has not become so commonplace. While there are a quite a number of providers using different protocols and equipment, FCEs have not entered into the day-to-day language of our largest healthcare provider, the NHS.

There are some different definitions of FCE, but one that is simple to understand and does not infer a particular healthcare system is

'primarily a measure of activity and activity limitation or occupational performance of a client, that is used to make recommendations for participation in work or the worker role while considering the person's impairment, environment and other influencing factors.' (Gibson & Strong 2003)

FCE aims to:

- Identify what your client can do
- Identify his or her capability of returning to work
- Determine work tolerance and endurance
- Provide an objective baseline for RTW planning
- Establish safe physical demand levels for future work (Raptosh 2005)

Generally speaking, the agency referring a person for an FCE would need to have specific questions answered, such as:

- Can my employee return to their own job?
- What sort of planned, phased RTW programme would be appropriate?

Table 2.10 Physical demand characteristics of work.

Physical demand level	Occasional 0–33% of the workday	Frequent 34–66% of the workday	Constant 67–100% of the workday	Typical energy required (METS)
Sedentary	10 lb	Negligible	Negligible	1.5–2.1
Light	20 lb	10 lb and/or walk/stand/ push/pull of arm/leg controls	Negligible and/or push/pull of arm/leg controls while seated	2.2–3.5
Medium	20–50 lb	10–25 lb	10 lb	3.6–6.3
Heavy	50–100 lb	25–50 lb	10–20 lb	6.4–7.5
Very heavy	> 100 lb	> 50 lb	> 20 lb	> 7.5

Leonard N Matheson, 1993

- What are the limiting factors for my patient in carrying out their job tasks?
- How much of an 8-hour day can my patient work?

The more specific the question, the more appropriately the FCE can be designed for your client. It is appropriate to carry out an FCE after a work-related injury, for short or long-term disabilities, before vocational retraining or career counselling (Raptosh 2005).

FCE has been developed to assess the physical activities associated with work, for instance walking, sitting or bending (Table 2.10). The evaluation of psychological and cognitive demands of a job does not seem so well developed. Traditionally, cognition, in terms of traumatic or acquired brain injury, has been assessed using neuropsychological tests to determine discrete functional difficulties. But this may be of limited use unless you can identify the cognitive job demands against which to match test results. This is a limitation of the FCE.

Mental residual functional capacity assessment
The Mental Residual Functional Capacity Assessment (Form SSA-4734-F4-SUP) in the USA is a measure used in social security claims. It looks at the claimant's ability to perform the functions they need for employment in spite of their disability. Each mental activity is evaluated within the context of the individual's capacity to sustain that activity over a normal working day and working week. The general areas are titled:

- Understanding and memory (three measures)
- Sustained concentration and persistence (eight measures)
- Social interaction (five measures)
- Adaptation (four measures)

The social security examiner may request this form, as may a hearings judge, or an attorney representing the applicant at the hearings stage of the appeal process. It is completed by a medical professional who has to back up their opinions with objective data Although this is not a functional capacity evaluation per se, it is one of the closest matched processes that could be found to date. It seems that this is an underdeveloped area in FCEs, and as common mental health problems are one of the most frequent reasons for sickness absence, it would seem timely to research this area more thoroughly.

There is no requirement to have a certificate of competence in carrying out FCE to date. However, one needs to have knowledge of neuromuscular systems, biomechanics, kinesiology, behavioural sciences and knowledge about adaptation of behaviour and environments. Courses and training are readily available in the USA and some training opportunities are now being made more widely available in the UK. Courses differ in how they are delivered – some are self-study while others require attendance at a study centre. They typically involve about 36 hours tuition. No one profession can lay claim to being the best choice to conduct an FCE. Often in the USA, an occupational therapist might carry out an FCE, with interdisciplinary co-operation from a physiotherapist and a psychologist.

Work tolerance
- How much work will I be able to do?
- Will I be able to tolerate an eight-hour day?
- Will I know if I have overdone it?

These are work tolerance questions that I have been asked and frankly found difficult to answer with any certainty. I am sure I am not alone. Another way of looking at work tolerance is using specific protocols to measure the cardiovascular output during exercise. This might be especially important in jobs with a high cardiovascular demand; when your client has cardiovascular deficits; or when your client has had a prolonged period of inactivity.

MET (metabolic equivalents of oxygen consumption) testing is currently used as a normal part of cardiovascular services and can be used at a submaximal level when following particular protocols such as the treadmill test (Modified Bruce Protocol), the Balke substandard treadmill test and the bench step test.

Submaximal MET testing is based on the concept that we can measure energy consumption by the volume of oxygen (VO_2) that a person consumes. There is a linear relationship between oxygen consumption and heart rate and as a workload increases the heart rate will increase in response. The submaximal MET test uses a protocol to predict the VO_{2max} in a safe manner to within 10–20% of the actual maximum level. The protocols provide a measure of the progressive workloads while the clinician assesses their client's heart rate. This process should only be carried out following specific training and with medical clearance of the treating physician. With regards to return to work, once the submaximal MET has been established, this can be correlated with the physical demand characteristics of work chart (Matheson 1993), which shows the typical energy required at the sedentary level through to the very heavy physical demand level over a typical eight-hour working day (Table 2.10).

FCE equipment
Different pieces of equipment are used to:

- Replicate work actions, for example, bend from the floor to a 50 cm shelf or lift 5 kg boxes
- Simulate work tasks, for example, holding a large heavy sack to simulate a sheep before shearing!

Different equipment will also be used depending on:

- the *type* of FCE, i.e:
  - o Matheson system
  - o Key functional assessment
  - o Blankenship FCE
  - o Isernhagen FCE
  - o BTE (Baltimore Therapeutic Equipment)
  - o JOULE System FCE by VALPAR International
- the *protocols* used, i.e:
  - o A set standardised system versus a flexible system based on individual needs
  - o The type of work a client does
  - o The individual client

You will usually need a fair amount of space to include all aspects of an FCE – approximately 40 × 40 metres. However, I have conducted FCEs in smaller clinic areas (approximately 8 × 8 metres) and then used the local community to do hill walks, steps and distance walking. The only problem in doing this is the weather sometimes and the obvious lack of control over the environment! You will need to decide whether a very controlled environment is what you require.

Table 2.11 shows some potentially useful pieces of equipment that can be sourced easily in or from the UK. Most of the standard pieces of equipment are fairly expensive, running into thousands of pounds, while non-standardised equipment tends to be much cheaper – in the tens to hundreds of pounds.

After an FCE, a report is usually written which, if conducted outside the litigation process, is primarily for the client, but can be shared with other parties, if the client agrees. The information gathered in the FCE is written in descriptive terms to:

- Compare the client's current ability with what their job demands of them.
- Answer the questions asked at the time of referral, for example, can Mr Smith return to his normal work duties?
- Indicate a plan of intervention or workplace restrictions, if appropriate.

Table 2.11 Potential functional capacity evaluation equipment.

Equipment	Selection of suppliers	Used for	Available from
Hand dynamometer	North Coast Medical (Promedics Ltd)	Designed to give reliable precise grip-force readings	www.promedics.co.uk
	Nottingham Rehab Supplies		www.nrs-uk.co.uk
Crawford small parts dexterity test	Harcourt Assessment	Assesses hand-eye co-ordination and fine motor dexterity	www.harcourt-uk.com
VCWS 1 – small tools (mechanical)	VALPAR International	Assesses the ability to make precise finger and hand movements and to work with small tools in tight or awkward spaces	www.valparint.com
Bennett hand tool dexterity test	Harcourt Assessment	Constructed to provide a measure of proficiency in using ordinary mechanics tools	www.harcourt-uk.com
VCWS 9 – whole body range of motion	VALPAR International	Assesses whole body range of motion, agility, and stamina through gross body movements of the trunk, arms, hands, legs, and fingers	www.valparint.com
VCWS 8 – simulated assembly	VALPAR International	Assesses the ability to perform repetitive assembly work requiring manipulation and bilateral use of the upper extremities	www.valparint.com
VCWS 19 – dynamic physical capacities	VALPAR International	Assesses various physical capacities while simulating work of a shipping and receiving clerk	www.valparint.com
General clerical test revised	Harcourt Assessment	Assess clerical speed and accuracy, numerical and verbal ability	www.harcourt-uk.com
Steps (wooden or exercise type)	Nottingham Rehab Supplies	To look at mobility on steps and tolerance to using steps	www.nrs-uk.co.uk
	A good fitness supplier		

Table 2.11 *continued.*

Equipment	Selection of suppliers	Used for	Available from
Heart rate monitor	BHIP Ltd Most high street department stores or a fitness supplier	Monitors basic information about how their bodies react during exercise	www.heartratemonitor.co.uk
Treadmill	Nottingham Rehab Supplies A good fitness supplier	To look at tolerance to walking and running	
Ladder – A-frame and straight	A good office supplier	Used for climbing and tolerance to climbing	
Lifting equipment EPIC lift capacity PILE lift box **Non-standardised Strong shelves**	Roy Matheson Inc. USA A good office supplier for a robust shelving unit	To simulate lifting and loading or to measure lifting and carrying capacity NB There is a certification course to undertake for the EPIC, which is on top of the cost of the equipment	www.roymatheson.com
Exercise weights	A good fitness supplier	Disc weights (as used in weight lifting) for use with a PILE lift box and job simulation	
Matheson bench	Roy Matheson Inc. USA	Primarily a positional tolerance device, it provides the opportunity for distraction-based observation of upper extremity dexterity, co-ordination, stooping/crouching and cognitive abilities	www.roymatheson.com
PrimusRS-work simulator	Baltimore Therapeutic Equipment (BTE) Distributed in the UK by	A combined unit that allows for duplicating hundreds of real-world job and daily living functions	Managed Medical Care Ltd, St Michael's House, Diss Business Park, Diss, Norfolk, IP22 4GT

Job simulation

Jacobs (1991) explains that many standardised and non-standardised assessment instruments have been developed, but none that are applicable to all populations. For this reason, she goes on to say that many occupational therapists (and possibly other professionals) have developed their own non-standardised assessments specifically for the population they work with. Nadeau and Buckheit (1995) say when referring to individuals who sustained a brain injury that:

> 'These (standardised) evaluation tools are not always reliable measures of cognitive function . . . particularly evident when assessing executive functions.'

One of the reasons given for this is that tests cannot answer all the questions that arise in clinical practice and their relevance to real-life situations. Nadeau and Buckheit (1995) go on to advocate job simulation as a feasible option to address these issues.

Work or job simulation is by its nature non-standardised, but inherently has more face validity for the client and therapist. While non-standardised, they can be designed in a structured and coherent manner with checks built in to ensure a robust process. The goal of this type of job simulation is different to that where it may be used as part of pre-employment screening in a recruitment and selection process. In the area of vocational rehabilitation one would usually be looking at many people and many different jobs. Job simulation is about re-creating the critical job demands to observe how a person copes with undertaking these. It can also provide the forum for role-playing difficult workplace situations that are seen as problematic for your client. Job simulations can be designed, therefore, to investigate a whole range of physical, psychological and emotional issues that might be present in a workplace and can be used for assessment or rehabilitation.

To carry out a realistic job simulation, it seems appropriate to first carry out a worksite assessment to gather information about the job demands and the environment itself. The armed forces have a well-established tradition of using their own designed job simulations to replicate the job demands and stresses of their particular type of work.

Simulations are often time-consuming to design and set up, but can reveal subtle detail about your client's functional abilities that other forms of testing might overlook, such as nuances in lifting particular items specific to the workplace or the interpersonal skills relating to a particular workplace meeting. They are seen as a safer alternative to exposing your client to a real-life situation. Well designed, they can also be used on an ongoing basis as part of rehabilitation with performance reviewed along the way. You may want to think about how best to rate your clients' performance and how you will encourage them to rate themselves before and after. Self-rating can be a useful approach with any client who finds it difficult to think ahead how their performance might meet the aim of the tasks.

Some clients might benefit from having their peer group rate them as well as a 'professional'. Rehab UK (www.rehabuk.org) is a charitable company that successfully uses peer groups in programmes with adults who have acquired brain injuries. Your current service design may restrict how flexible you can be with job simulation and it may be useful to reflect on whether this is limiting your clients in how they are assessed. Would peer groups be more beneficial than one-to-one sessions? Is job simulation more appropriate than the traditional testing more frequently used?

If there are key pieces of equipment that your client normally handles, such as computer software, paperwork, boxes and tools, personal protective equipment (PPE) such as hard hat, gloves and overalls, this will all add to the perceived relevancy of the assessment.

> With our case study John (p. 19) if we set up a simulation of a work task to assess his functional ability in moving shopping trolleys about a car park, there would be less face validity using a wheelchair indoors on a linoleum floor compared with a real trolley, outside in a car park, with John wearing his usual constrictive PPE. If John had concerns about dealing with an angry member of the public, this would require some careful scripting and acting in relation to angry situations that are likely to happen in a supermarket car park – not confrontations in a doctor's surgery, for instance.

If you have a client group with similar vocational concerns you might find it worthwhile to design and construct several job simulations to address a range of functional abilities, for instance:

- A production line with fine finger movements and reaching – to help to assess work-related upper limb pain and difficulty making repetitive movements
- An office situation with increasing numbers and types of distractions – to assess difficulties with concentration and the skills to cope with this situation
- A healthcare setting where patient moving and handling causes back pain and where the patient can be replaced by objects or another willing volunteer – to assess safe body mechanics and handling techniques

As with all assessments, client safety is paramount and risk assessment should be integral to the design of any simulations. The assessor should also act within their scope of practice to ensure safe and ethical practice. You may want to hire an experienced health and safety officer or another professional to design your job simulations.

Job matching
One of the most important aspects of vocational rehabilitation is the process of job matching – obtaining a good fit between a job and the person doing the job. This concept affects everyone who works, not just your clients. It affects you, too. Job matching is not based wholly on the physical or psychological aspects of job demands. It also includes the workplace environment, encompassing its physical environment and the workplace culture, social politics, procedures and policies.

Job matching lies at the heart of the supported employment model – Leach (2002) says:

> 'The process of job matching at its most basic level is that of comparing the information from the client's vocational profile with the characteristics of an available job, as outlined in the job analysis, and then detailing the way in which you will try to bridge the gaps between the two.'

Like other aspects of assessment in vocational rehabilitation, job matching has a cyclical pattern. You might have to reassess more than once and try a few similar jobs before you are successful in obtaining a good fit. To build up a vocational profile with a client, job tasters may be used. This can be especially useful if your client has never worked, or if they have to make a radical change in direction. Job tasters are a useful method for situational assessment that is an assessment of real life over a period of time. The methods used would normally be a combination of self-rating, peer observation and rating and or behavioural observations. Different services may have developed their own particular assessment forms for this and usually they require the client to self-rate their abilities. However, it would be possible to use your assessment results to add into this process – this can be helpful if your client has difficulty stating their own abilities realistically.

Summary

In all of this process, it is essential that you build up clear lines of communication up with employers to facilitate the process. The employer needs to feel as confident as your client coming into the workplace. Ignorance breeds suspicion and knowledge is power. So ensure that you set aside time within your assessment process to spend with the employer to educate them about your client and your assessment processes – and be ready to do all this on the hop. If your employer is a small enterprise, it is likely that there will be considerable demands on his or her time. You might want to suggest a breakfast meeting or an early evening meeting to suit the employer.

Career-based assessments

The purpose of career assessments is to provide an insight into the career decisions that a person has made to date and those decisions they have yet to take. Assessments will normally cover areas of interest to your client, the current transferable skills that they have and the local job market. The assessments themselves will most heavily rely on the narrative your client will tell you about him or herself. They may also include psychometric testing and psychometric questionnaires (personality trait types, for instance). The goal is to facilitate the client to see him or herself as marketable – looking at transferable skills that are relevant now and in the future and to consider aspects of lifelong learning to remain in work.

Some people assume that if someone is struggling with their current occupation, they need to move their career downwards to a 'less demanding' job. However, the solution is never as straightforward or as simple as this. Japp (2005) explains that our social life often revolves around work, friends are from work and we describe ourselves by the job that we do. Our social status is often a reflection of the job we do. To take on a 'less demanding' job can suggest a less prestigious role. It is unsurprising, therefore, if downsizing in this manner is not always met with enthusiasm.

A more positive way forward is to adopt the supported employment approach of acknowledging that:

> 'Individuals with disabilities know what is best for them and the support strategy needs to reflect their input, aspirations and dreams.' (Leach 2002)

Career theories

It is often helpful to base your assessments on particular theories as they can provide some structure and methods to interpret data. Since the early 20th century there have been career theories that help to explain why people make the career choices they do and attempt to provide strategies for this process of career decision making. There are too many career theories to name in this book. Textbooks that address this topic adequately include Brown and Brooks (1996) and Sharf (1992). One drawback of many of the career theories is that they were developed to explain work and work behaviour associated with white European males. Having said that, John Holland's work on trait factor theory has been extensively researched worldwide and Beckett and Betz's Social Cognitive Career Theory (SCCT) also has a diverse research population.

John Holland developed his trait theory because he saw career choice as an extension of a person's personality and that we seek to find a 'fit' between the work environment and ourselves (Sharf 1992). We seek to define our vocational choices in terms of stable personality traits and then adapt our behaviour to achieve

> 'satisfaction, stability and performance.' (Brown & Brooks 1996)

So behaviour is determined by an interaction between personal traits and the environment. The assessment tool that has been developed for this theory is the Self-directed Search (SDS)(www.self-directed-search.com) The assessment has a variety of forms, including an audio version. It is available in a range of languages, versions for different educational levels and an online version. It takes approximately 45 minutes to carry out and this can be done individually or in a group.

It is a useful assessment tool because it offers information immediately on what types of work environment might suit a particular personality type. It is relatively simple to see where there might be poor person–environment fit for a client. This can add another dimension to your overall assessment and may give clues to the obstacles in the progress of a person's return to work.

The SCCT emphasises the importance of cognition, learning and self-direction in career development. Rather than a fixed idea of personality type, this theory proposes that people have the ability to change and recognises the influence of external and internal barriers in career decision making. Lent et al. base the SCCT on the social cognitive perspective – in particular Albert Bandura's work – and developed it in the late 1980s and early 1990s (Savickas & Lent 1994; Brown & Brooks 1996). The SCCT focuses on the interaction of personal goals, outcome expectations and self-efficacy on choices made about careers. The critical components are associated with the expected success and the valued compensation an individual feels about their choices. Contextual factors influence the individual's perception about his or her ability to succeed. If barriers are perceived as significant, this leads to weaker interest and choice actions.

To date, I have not been able to find an assessment tool for the SCCT similar to the SDS for Holland's theory. However, if you become familiar with the theory (and self-efficacy in particular) you can apply the theoretical reasoning to the narrative that you will obtain from your assessment with your client. The idea is to identify levels of interest and some personal goals and then to investigate the barriers that your client perceives as interfering with achieving their personal career goals.

Transferable skills

Whichever career theory you choose to adopt, you are still advised to address transferable skills when working with someone who may want to make a career change.

Your client may not feel able or comfortable returning to their old job as a consequence of the time off sick. If this is the case, or if you are seeing someone who has not worked for a while or never worked, they will need to know how to identify their own current transferable work skills and how they can add new transferable skills to their repertoire to engage in work.

Transferable skills may not just be those historically used in the workplace such as fitting double glazing. They include those skills used on a daily basis and not necessarily recognised as useful to a work environment, such as clear verbal communication, welcoming demeanour and managing a household budget successfully. To help your client identify their transferable skills, you can facilitate him or her to focus on their perceived abilities and current skills.

Several texts refer to skills or transferable skills as strengths associated with an individual. (Leach 2002; Blesedell Crepeau et al. 2003; Marchington & Wilkinson 2003; Japp 2005). However, the organisation of these skills is varied and if you are new to transferable skills, it may be helpful to have a structure to help you and your client look at his or her skills.

The UK Government website says:

'Literacy, language and numeracy skills cover the ability to read, write and speak English or Welsh and to use mathematics at a level that enables you to function and progress at work and society in general. Key skills are similar but include a wider range of skills.' (www.direct.gov.uk)

The Government's six key skills are:

1. Communication
2. Information technology
3. Working with numbers
4. Working with others
5. Problem solving
6. Improving your own learning and performance

I would like to add physical and functional skills to this list.

Career decision making skills and transitions

Accessing specialist careers advice and assessment in the UK can be made through a variety of Government opportunities. To keep up to date, I advise you to access those services that have responsibility for education and training and job searching and placements. As contracts and policy are ever changing you would be wise to contact your local providers to establish which parts of their services are free and which might demand a fee – and who should pay this fee (for example, the client or Jobcentre Plus). If you are not au fait with the services of your client's local community, I encourage you to make the time to investigate this. In the long run you will probably avoid unnecessary duplication of services, which is costly. Some current useful websites are:

UK Government   (www.direct.gov.uk)
Worktrain   (www.worktrain.gov.uk)

National jobs and learning website with information and advice on childcare and voluntary work

Jobcentre or Jobcentre Plus   (www.jobcentreplus.gov.uk)

Can help your client find work and get careers advice

Connexions   (www.connexions-direct.com)

Help with career choice

Department for Education and Skills   (www.dfes.gov.uk)

Established with the purpose of creating opportunity, releasing potential and achieving excellence for all.

One model of career decision making is seen in Figure 2.3

Self-awareness Knowing one's aptitudes and skills Positive self-concept and self-esteem Knowing one's values, interests and needs Self-efficacy and belief in self Maturity and responsibility Knowing the importance of one's own roles
Opportunity awareness Access to information about training and work opportunities Choice and decision-making about overcoming barriers to work Support from family/carers/others Self-awareness and opportunity awareness lead to
Career decision making The vocational counsellor's role is to support the client through this process of transition and to develop a life management plan

Figure 2.3 A career decision-making process.
McDonald R (1996–97), Deaking University, Australia.

Environment-based assessments

Environment-based assessments provide information about the work tasks and the environment in which they happen. The assessments can also provide information about the environment (communities) in which a person travels to get to work. Assessments might occur inside the workplace, looking at the job tasks, the internal and the external aspects of the work environment. It is widely recognised that assessing an individual in the environment in which they intend to work gives the most realistic picture but it also should be appreciated that this ideal is not always possible. Influences such as health and safety issues, the wishes of the client, the manager, the health practitioner and the family, the service constraints that the assessor works under may prevent the assessor going into a workplace. This is specifically addressed in Function-based assessments (p. 40).

The aspects of the environment that you will ultimately assess will depend on the needs that you and your client have explored and those priorities that have been agreed. The goals of the assessments are to identify and describe the demands that a job places on an individual and to evaluate the potential obstacles. The assessments should facilitate you and your client to identify which tasks are likely to be difficult to carry out and why and to start to consider the solutions. Environment-based assessments will be subdivided into: worksite assessments, job analyses, work study, health and safety and travel to work. You will (in the most part) be entering a workplace on the invitation of the employer and as such should

Table 2.12 Seen and unseen elements in a workplace.

Seen elements	Unseen elements
Policies	Workplace culture
Tools and equipment	Attitudes
Other employees	Politics
Procedures	Pressure/stress
Safety	Hierarchy
Cleanliness	
Processes of working	
Productivity	
Job descriptions	
Organisational structure	

After Handy (1993) *Understanding Organisations*, 4th edn

conduct your proceedings with respect and professionalism whatever your personal feelings. It is of utmost importance that there is clear communication between the people conducting the assessments to engender confidence not only in you and your service but also the process of return to work that you recommend.

The workplace itself is a combination of the seen and unseen elements as listed in Table 2.12 and some or all of these can be part of environment-based assessments related to vocational rehabilitation and your clients' needs. A number of professions may be involved to assess the workplace and identify those issues pertinent to your client, e.g. health and safety officer, ergonomist or work psychologist.

Environment-based assessments inherently address issues to do with the surroundings but do include many human aspects such as culture, attitudes and your client's work colleagues. Haglund and Henriksson (1995) cited in Sandqvist and Henriksson (2004) divide the work environment into two aspects that can be a helpful way of understanding workplace issues and obstacles.

- The occupational *norm* – the sociocultural consensus on how an activity should be carried out
- The occupational *circumstances* – environmental attributes and demands necessary to carry out an activity

In terms of return to work, environment-based assessments are used to help identify work-related barriers or obstacles with your client. The 'flags' system (Table 2.9) is a way of categorising the issues pertinent in return to work. They highlight the common issues that are obstacles in return to work. Blue flags are those work-related obstacles (Main & Burton 2000) that include worker-specific perceptions about the relationship between injuries and working, blame, perceived work demands and the psychosocial aspects of work. Black flags, as described by Main and Burton (2000), are those obstacles external to the person *'being more characteristics of the occupational environment, and all workers in a given setting may be equally exposed.' (Health and Safety Executive (HSE) 2005)*

Black flags involve local organisational constraints and can include organisational policy and procedures. They also include actual practice reflecting employer's perceptions and attitudes about such issues as sickness certification, modified work and concerns over early return to work (HSE 2005).

These types of environment-based assessments are also known as worksite assessments, job analyses, ergonomic assessments, and job site analysis. Many different people will already carry out assessments in the workplace as part of their jobs. For instance:

- *Occupational health and safety officer* – worksite assessment based around understanding the environmental hazards
- *Human resources* – job analyses in relation to recruitment
- *Engineers* – detailed studies of new manufacturing processes to identify risks to the workforce

So it is helpful to be absolutely sure that everyone understands what the intention of your assessment is, so that misinterpretations are minimised.

Worksite assessments

The organisation
There may be elements associated with the organisation that would help in planning a person's return to work. These can include:

- Understanding the purpose of the organisation (the business aspects)
- What the organisation produces to sell
- The organisational structure and hierarchy
- The policies and procedures affecting your client returning to work (or being recruited)
- The workplace politics and culture

Structure and hierarchy
The structure of an organisation can give a sense of the flow of information and communication channels. A very flat organisational structure may allow a range of people to take responsibilities and make decisions, whereas a triangular structure may have very few people at the top of the triangle who make decisions and take responsibility. This has obvious implications when you are attempting to get permission from an organisation to do a worksite assessment or take photographs or decide when your client can return to work. Only a few people in an organisation traditionally make financial decisions – and getting to know who they are can help you save time, for instance when you are negotiating who will pay for a new adjustable office chair.

Policies and procedures

Understanding the work routines can help in the design of a return to work plan. Working hours, shift patterns, breaks and types of work are all important information.

Work practices and how things are conducted add further detail. Policies and procedures help to give some structure to what happens in an organisation. If you are working with an employer who has written policies and procedures, then asking to see them or discussing them with human resources or a manager can help to explain how to help your client return to work. If the employer does not have anything written down, there may well be a tradition of doing things a certain way. In this instance the person who has been working there the longest may be able to shed some light on how a return to work has been previously managed.

If the workplace has written job descriptions, these can shed light on the major components of the job such as the roles and responsibilities and lines of communication and authority. They may describe actual duties and the level of training and personal aptitudes that are required to carry out the work. However, many employees do not have job descriptions and even fewer self-employed people will have.

It is important to be aware of the support services that an organisation may have access to internally and externally. Some larger organisations have access to occupational health services (with an occupational health physician and nurse), some may have occupational health advisors who may have some qualifications in health and safety, there should be a health and safety officer and there may be union representation on staff. Some employers will operate an employee assistance programme (EAP) offering confidential 24/7 telecare, i.e. counselling and advice over the telephone or face-to-face interventions. It normally would include counselling for a range of concerns such as money, bullying or domestic violence, and some EAPs will also provide welfare advice.

Employee health insurance is something else to ask about – this may be able to offer some rehabilitation interventions such as physiotherapy or chiropractic. Likewise, enquiring about employers' insurance policies (such as employers liability or personal accident) may reveal support for your client's return to work rehabilitation, as might the income protection insurance policies that some self-employed people have.

Workplace politics and culture

Policies and procedures usually only give part of the picture. The workplace culture can have a strong influence on the people working in a particular place but is often the hardest to pin down. One might 'get a feeling' that might be accepting and positive or suspicious and negative when carrying out an assessment but nothing substantial enough to document successfully. However, the general behaviours and attitudes in a workplace can be the make or break of a return to work. *'The way we do things around here'* is a common definition of organisational culture. It refers to the shared values, beliefs and assumptions in a workplace. It is about feeling as if you belong. Charles Handy has written a number of books on this topic and further details about organisational culture can be found in his texts such as *Understanding Organisations* (1993).

Understanding the workplace culture can be particularly important to those clients who find it difficult to read subtle non-verbal communication and who find it confusing trying to understand complex social behaviours. Common questions that can yield interesting answers are:

- 'How does your workplace treat people who have been off sick?'
- 'What do you and your colleagues think of people who take time off sick?'

Supporting your client closely during the return to work phase can be one way to recognise and deal with unhelpful issues to do with organisational culture and help your client to cope.

Have you ever worked in a place where you just didn't feel like you fit?

What did you do to try and blend in and feel comfortable?

What could you learn from this experience to help your client?

The worksite environment

In addressing the worksite, this text will not attempt to cover the broad topic of ergonomics, as there are many others that describe this professional area eminently well. Ergonomics can be defined as

> '*the scientific study of human beings in relation to their working environments.*' *(Pheasant 1986, cited in Hagedorn 2000)*

A second definition explains that ergonomics is

> '*the scientific study of people at work and the work system within which they operate.*' *(Stuckey & Meyer 2000)*

Much of what is mentioned in this text can therefore be seen under the title of ergonomics.

In the physical environment, one would expect to take note of and in some instances make measurements of the factors seen in Table 2.13. These factors are taken into consideration because of the potential hazardous effects they may have on an individuals. If you are not experienced or suitably qualified to assess these environmental aspects yourself, then it is important to identify who could make an assessment with you. You may need to call in the expertise of a noise consultant, or a lighting expert or an industrial hygienist to help. Some of the basic tools that may of help to most vocational rehabilitation practitioners would be:

Table 2.13 Factors to consider in a worksite assessment.

Environmental factor	Potential effect
Ranges of temperatures, humidity	Acclimatisation effects, task performance reduction
	Physiological changes
	Reduced mobility due to protective clothing
Noise (continuous and sudden)	Discomfort in the ears and hearing loss (temporary and permanent)
Lighting/illumination	Discomfort and eyestrain
	Difficulty in seeing tasks
Exposure to weather conditions	Effects are similar to those of temperatures, humidity and noise
Air quality and circulation	Breathing and visual difficulties due to dust or smoke for instance
	Circulated air can help to reduce ambient temperatures
Flooring	Flooring types can affect tolerance to static standing, noise reduction and hygiene.
Cleanliness and tidiness	Debris around a worksite can be a tripping hazard
	Cleanliness affects the hygiene in a workplace
Substances (toxic and non-toxic)	Effects can range from discomfort or difficulty carrying tasks to physiological harm e.g. chemical burns
Smells	General discomfort and some difficulty concentrating on tasks
Electricity	Hazard for burns and electrocution
	Wires on the floor or strung up can be a tripping and falling hazard
Mechanical hazards	Machinery can cause entrapment if not sufficiently guarded includes automatic doors
Radiations	Ultraviolet, X-ray, radioactive radiations can have potentially harmful effects as they can penetrate the body's skin defences
	Particular hazard in pregnancy
General maintenance of building fabric	Potential of falling debris from poorly maintained buildings
Gradients	Slopes up and down can provide slipping hazards
Vibration	General discomfort, disruption of visual acuity, tickling sensations. These effects can be negative to motivation and also cause task degradation
	Extreme exposure can lead to permanent physiological changes such as vibration white finger

- tape measure (20m +)
- light meter
- gradiometer
- digital camera/video

Job analysis

Job analysis can be explained as

'an analytical process designed to collect data about jobs.' (Lysaght 1996)

Analysing jobs into their constituent parts started in the 1930s in the USA as a result of massive job losses in the economic depression of the time. US Congress at the time initiated the first employee assistance programme and also started research into occupations. Thus was born the first edition of the *Dictionary of Occupational Titles* (DOT), which aimed to provide a comprehensive listing of all occupations in the USA and provide reliable descriptions of the work that was required to match people to jobs. It also served to provide a uniform language so that there was less individual interpretation of each occupational title such as 'joiner' or 'engineer'. In more recent publications, the DOT has also identified the relevant skills and training required to perform the occupations and this has all been achieved through job analyses. Miller et al. (1980) reported that 75 000 onsite job analyses were conducted to produce the fourth edition of the DOT, which describes 28 800 occupational titles!

Lysaght (1997) explains that a vast body of knowledge exists in industrial and organisational psychology, industrial engineering and kinesiology related to job analysis. Human resources departments use job analyses within their day-to-day work. *Role analysis* may be a more accurate term to use for this professional group as their job analyses focus on the content of a job to provide a useful description for the organisation itself, i.e. building up job descriptions and person specifications (Marchington & Wilkinson 2003). In relation to vocational rehabilitation, job analysis is more concerned with integrating disabled people and those people with illnesses into work and the workplace. Fransisco Canelón (1995) states:

'When clinical reasoning indicates a good rehabilitation potential, a job site analysis is conducted to determine the essential functions of the client's work.'

During the late 20th century the DOT was replaced by the O*NET classification and analysis system (http://online.onetcenter.org) and this has been based on occupational keywords rather than job titles (primarily for use by the US Employment Service). However, the DOT remains in existence in paper and electronic formats (www.occupationalinfo.org). O*NET

'reflects the character of occupations (via job-oriented descriptors) and people (via worker-oriented descriptors). The Content Model also allows occupational

information to be applied across jobs, sectors, or industries (cross-occupational descriptors) and within occupations (occupational-specific descriptors).' (www.theodora.com/new/onet.html)

Considering that job analyses have been carried out for over six decades, there remains no absolute way of conducting one. This assessment is not owned by any one profession and each puts its own philosophical slant on the process. Lysaght (1997) explains that there is agreement generally that a job analysis involves the breakdown of jobs by knowledge, skills, abilities, behaviours or by worker accountability.

Organising and carrying out a job analysis

The literature generally does not describe specific processes to explain how to carry out a job analysis but there will be a need to observe the job in question at some stage. You can expect to be quite physically active in a job analysis, following people around who are working, seeing what they are doing and asking lots of questions. You may want to get permission to photograph or video particular work tasks so enable a more detailed analysis to happen later. You may want to fill in a form, use a checklist, a questionnaire or to take notes as you go around a work-site. You may need some tools to take with you, such as a stopwatch to measure repetitions or cycles of tasks, or a tape measure to measure working spaces. You may also want to review certain organisational policies and procedures about return to work, job descriptions or accident reports or sickness records. It will depend on the actual focus of your assessment based on your client's particular needs. For instance, you would not need to look at the sickness absence record an employer keeps in every case.

There are potential difficulties with job analyses, and Lysaght (1997) warns about the overdependence on checklists and forms as these can oversimplify the complex nature of work and workplaces. An analysis is time-consuming if done in adequate detail, and while every client would benefit from this assessment, a service provider will need to account for this both in terms of finances and staff resources. One difficulty with analysing jobs that do not involve a wide range of physical postures is capturing the cognitive and perceptual elements sufficiently. Another recognised complexity is when people work in a team model where everyone takes responsibility for all the tasks to be accomplished and where job tasks vary widely over time, be that over a day, a month or over a season.

Seasonal differences are particularly evident in the farming industry where certain activities, such as harvesting crops or weaning young animals occur at certain times of the season, and this poses a problem in capturing all the essential activities that someone may have to do. Two recognised approaches for analysing jobs are Fleishman's Ability Requirements Scale (Fleishman & Mumford 1991) and Farrell's Fine Detailed Work and Action Posture code (Farrell & Littlejohn 1999). Both of these approaches could provide useful tools for structuring and carrying out job analyses.

Bearing in mind your own role in your service, what information would be useful to you that you might gain from a job analysis?

The following description is just one way of organising and conducting job analyses and it is based on a blend of my own experiences and insights from colleagues and published papers. I have, wherever possible, cited original authors. Personally, I like to spend some time explaining the purpose of the job analysis and how it relates to an individual and the return to work and rehabilitation. There will be some work on the assessor's part that can be done ahead of visiting a workplace that will help to describe the job in detail, such as describing the steps involved in each task, and identifying which tasks need to be done in a team. Scheduling a meeting before the worksite visit can be used to discuss these points also. Organising ahead of time is key to obtaining information in as efficient a manner as possible. After gathering basic information about the organisation, the supervisors, and the environment, the job analysis per se can begin.

Ellexson (1997) describes the following components to consider in a job analysis:

- Essential and marginal job tasks
- Work activity analysis
- Frequency/time spent
- Measurements
- Environmental considerations
- Working alone/teams
- Degree of skill required
- Physical requirements
- Cognitive considerations
- Psychological requirements
- Physiological considerations

It is necessary to determine the job role and the key (essential) tasks that facilitate the success of the job because long gone are the days when an employer could afford to pay someone for not contributing towards the overall purpose of an organisation. Every job also has tasks that are required but are not essential to the role, for example:

- A software developer has to prepare invoices for his time, but this doesn't help to build programming code.
- A farmer has to complete statistical data about his farm, but this doesn't help the cows being milked.
- A line operative has to sweep up and empty bins but this doesn't result in more chocolates being packed.

Ellexson (1997) recommends taking each task and breaking them down further into the steps that are required (work activity analysis). Each task may involve repetitive cycles of movements and actions and these (frequencies) should ideally be measured in time using a stopwatch unless using a specific work study methodology. Several measurements will need to be taken to give a range and if several people do the same job, it can be useful to time different people. If time is not an issue in the job role, this element may not be required. Associated with this is how many times a task or action has to be repeated and how many people might be available to do a particular task. Linked to the measurements part of the job analysis are the environmental considerations that should be taken into account (Table 2.13).

Other measurements to consider are those concerning the space in which the task occurs. This is the detailed ergonomic part of the job analysis which weighs loads and measures:

- Pull and push forces (using a force gauge)
- Carrying distances
- Tool dimensions
- Work space

You will need to decide whether you have the skills to carry out these assessments or whether you need to engage an ergonomist to do this part of the job analysis. It is beyond the scope of this book to detail these processes – a text that may be helpful for therapists is Karen Jacobs' *Ergonomics for Therapists* (1991) (2nd edition). There are also training courses that can be taken at a number of British universities to postgraduate level to provide further qualifications, as well as independent providers of training. The Ergonomics Society (www.ergonomics. org.uk) in the UK is the body that ergonomists can join depending on the training they have received. The society has developed a framework for knowledge and competence and has a list of registered service providers who meet their own guidelines.

An important distinction to make about the tasks is whether they are carried out alone or as a team, sometimes or all the time. Team working has different social dynamics to working alone and motivation to work can differ, due to feelings of letting other people down because of reduced performance. Part of the job analysis will be to identify who is responsible for which tasks in team working and what happens if a team cannot perform their own tasks.

Whether a job or parts of a job require certain levels of skill or qualification is important to deduce to ensure that particular competencies are met prior to returning to work. This can be essential for the health and safety of everyone in the workplace.

Physical demands
The physical demands of tasks can be observed fairly easily and photos and video can assist a more detailed evaluation so that the assessor's memory is not relied

on totally. This can have the added benefit of reducing the amount of time spent on a worksite. A job demands questionnaire can be used to structure an interview when obtaining information about a job. However, this typically would address only the physical elements. Questions such as 'How often do you use a foot pedal?' or, 'How heavy are the loads you carry?' will be used to determine the physical demands of the work. A free copy of a job demands questionnaire can be obtained through the American Epic Rehab website at www.epicrehab.com. If your skills do not cover human functioning, then you may need to consider having an occupational therapist do this part of the assessment, as this is one of the core competencies in which this profession are trained.

Cognitive demands

The cognitive demands will be less easy to observe. Some deduction can be made from certain activities, such as talking on the telephone and writing down messages requiring sustained attention and divided attention, concentration, working memory and visual perception. Discussing the demands with workers and managers will also lend insight into the demands. It will be useful to have understanding of cognition and its components before attempting this area. You will need to decide whether you have the skills or whether you need the specialist services and skills of a work-based psychologist. Associated with cognition are the psychological or psychosocial considerations – these can include stressful elements in the workplace such as production standards or one's control over work tasks, responsibilities, work relationships and job satisfaction.

A job demands chart can be a useful tool to document these elements and to compare them alongside the functional abilities of your client to help to determine if there is a sufficient match or otherwise. Table 2.14 is an example of a job demands chart and a partially worked example for a joiner.

Physiological demands

Ellexson (1997) recommends looking at the physiological considerations of a job. These are the natural domain of the occupational health nurse and physician and pertain to the adverse effects a workplace can have on an individual's bodily functions. The workplace ill-health issues such as the effect of noise or radiation or heat on a person is vital in maintaining healthy working. Certain tasks that involve static postures can adversely affect blood pressure – for example, repetitive turning of a handle might contribute to wrist pain. While knowledge of human physiology is an advantage, unless you have specific occupational health training you are likely to require the skills of an occupational health nurse.

Figure 2.4 shows a worked example of a form used during a worksite visit to help in organising job analyses.

Reporting the data

Once the worksite assessment and job analysis have been conducted, the data needs to be compiled into a logical report. This will usually be carried out in conjunction with other assessments that will be pertinent to your client's situation. So

Table 2.14 Example job demands chart: worked example for a joiner.

	Demand of job determined by job analysis	Client's ability determined by assessment of client	Match?
Strength			
Lifting	Heavy from 0 to 1.70 m Occasional lifting cupboards onto a wall fitting	Lifting was tested to within the heavy physical demand level	Yes at the lower end
Carrying	Medium to heavy Occasional tool boxes, cupboards, building materials, etc.	Carrying was tested to the medium physical demand for 212½ feet. Ceased carrying due to pain	Yes for distances shorter than 200 feet and lighter weights
Pushing	Adjusting cupboards into spaces		
Pulling	As above		
Mobility			
Sitting	Up to 30 minutes, driving to a job or collecting materials	No difficulties noted	Yes
Dynamic standing	Constant All jobs requiring some standing and moving from foot to foot	No difficulties noted	Yes
Static standing	Occasional When fixing closures or sawing wood		
Walking	Occasional To collect items to carry	Tested on a ½ mile walk on the level and up/down cobbled streets No increase in symptoms reported	Yes
Agility			
Stairs/ladders	Stairs in clients' property Ladder use for roofing jobs and above head height work Occasional	6 flights of stairs with 10 steps on each flight No difficulties noted	Yes

Table 2.14 *continued.*

	Demand of job determined by job analysis	Client's ability determined by assessment of client	Match?
Balancing	Ladder work and working at heights, e.g. roofs Occasional	Not tested due to risk of falling (balance difficulties)	
Crouching/ kneeling	Reaching work low area Frequent	Tested and client complained of some knee discomfort No functional decline noted	Yes with discomfort
Stooping	Reaching work low area Occasional	Tested filling out paperwork Client complained of neck pain and ceased activity after approximately 10 minutes	Yes with discomfort
Bending	To pick up items Frequent	Tested in materials handling element Poor body mechanics noted	Yes with some tuition
Twisting/spinal rotation	Frequent and can include weights	Minor discomfort noted	Yes with discomfort
Above shoulder work	Reaching to fit cupboards, shelving, etc. Occasional	Repetitive reaching caused pain in his right upper arm	Yes with discomfort
Low level work	Reaching on a frequent basis	Losing balance when reaching low down	No
Dexterity			
Fine finger	Use of nails, screws and other ironmongery Frequent	Functional use of hands but demonstrated slowed speed	Yes if speed is not required
Grasp – light			
Grasp – firm			
Pinching			

Table 2.14 *continued.*

	Demand of job determined by job analysis	Client's ability determined by assessment of client	Match?
Writing			
Handling	Tool use, driving	Tested with results demonstrating functional use	Yes
Reaching upwards	Reaching to fit cupboards, shelving, etc. Occasional	Some increased pain in his right upper arm	Yes with discomfort
Reaching forwards	Reaching to fit cupboards, shelving, etc. Occasional	Some increased pain in his right upper arm	Yes with discomfort
Foot controls	Driving Occasional	Not tested	?
Coordination			
Eye-hand			
Eye-hand-foot			
Vision/hearing			
Visual perception	Driving, tool use, measuring etc. Constant	Not tested	?
Near acuity (< 20 inches)	Majority of detailed work		
Far acuity (> 20 ft)	Viewing rooms and buildings from afar		
Colour vision	Required to differentiate kitchen work surface choice of customer		
Depth perception	Required		
Hearing	Required		Partial
Cognition			

Table 2.14 *continued.*

	Demand of job determined by job analysis	**Client's ability determined by assessment of client**	**Match?**
Understanding instructions	Comprehension of what the client needs (verbally) Understanding written instructions from packs of materials Reading blueprints/plans Awareness of building regulations, local authority requirements etc. Occasional	Followed verbal and written instructions with minimal verbal cueing	No
Memory	Remembering how to construct objects, e.g. doorframes	Remembers how to build well-known items Struggles with new designs	
Concentration/ attention	Requires sustained attention, alternating attention and divided attention on tasks	Has a difficulty with auditory distractions Anger can flare in these situations	
Productivity			
Quantity	Self-paced but demands from customers	Produces less per hour than previously, therefore taking longer to finish jobs	Partial
Quality	High degree of quality Little margin for error from a safety and aesthetic point	Retains high quality of work	Yes
Attendance	Requires regular attendance until the job is complete		Yes
Timeliness	Requires punctual start and finish times		Yes
Safety			

Table 2.14 *continued.*

	Demand of job determined by job analysis	Client's ability determined by assessment of client	Match?
Adherence to safety rules			
Use of proper body mechanics			Yes
Use of protective behaviour		Uses old PPE	Partial
Interpersonal behaviour			
Response to supervision	N/A works alone		
Response to co-workers	N/A works alone		
Response to change	Jobs and locations change every few days	Anxious about driving to new location	Partial
Attitude to work/role	Requires a positive attitude as he is working directly with customers	Strong worker role identity and positive attitude to working	Yes

there may be information about functional abilities, physical strength and mental health. However, your report that describes the workplace should do exactly that – describe the workplace and the job that you have observed, discussed and measured. It is useful to take notes as you carry out your assessment and these (if legible) can form part of your own records system. Most workplaces would also expect to see some formal report following your assessment. If specific tests or protocols have been used during the assessments, these should be documented and the reason for their use explained, as this will form part of your clinical reasoning.

How the report is structured will rather depend on the purpose it serves and how much time as a practitioner you have to write down your findings formally. You can discuss this with the employer and your service manager. Some services will write a report detailing the problem areas and recommendations in an easy to read list format and other services will need to describe the work environment and the job analyses in detail. However you construct the report, you should follow your own profession's guidelines and best practice.

JOB ANALYSIS
JOB TASKS AND FUNCTIONAL DEMANDS
Client Name__John Brown__Ref:_NLD05het89____Date_21032006_

Employer Cosmos Dye Works	**Organisation's function** To dye fabrics for the clothing industry.
Manager Frank Le Blanc	**Director** Margery Ellwood
Current job title Engineering Technician	**Length of employment** 18 years
Job role To maintain the running of the machinery used in the dye works.	
Experience/training required (licences, tickets etc) Mechanical engineering qualification Forklift driving licence	
Skills required Able to work alone and set own workloads Sound engineering knowledge Literacy and numeracy Analysis skills Attention to detail and good time management Interpersonal skills with colleagues	
Line manager Steve Crow	**Human Resources** Alice Bottle
Occupational Health None available	**H&S** Fred Harris
Union rep N/A	**Union details** Amicus Union www.amicustheunion.org/
Hours of work 39 hours, Mon-Fri 6am to 2pm except Fri, finishes at 1pm	**Shift patterns** No
Pay £19 870	**Overtime/bonuses** none
Workplace support (health insurance, EAP, union etc) None Telephone advice from the union	
Works alone yes/~~no~~/~~sometimes~~ **Details** Is the only person who carries out all the tasks for this job. Works on site only	**Works in a team** ~~yes~~/no/~~sometimes~~ **Details**

Figure 2.4 Job tasks and functional demands.

Job description ~~yes~~/no	Contract of employment yes/~~no~~
Copied yes/no	

Essential tasks	Marginal tasks
Forklift driving to pick up containers and move around the site Running the water plant operations pH water checks Water hardness check Borehole water check Reservoir checks	Emptying industrial bins Sweeping floors to remove debris Fixing other plant machinery Health and safety assessments Legionnaires' risk assessment

Tools/equipment used
Forklift truck
Spanners/wrenches
Litmus paper
Pyrex specimen jars

Job task	Frequency	Physical demand	Psychological demand	Cognitive demand	Physiological demand
Running the water plant operations	Continuous, daily No other people do this job Each check takes 1 hour 15 minutes to complete	Walking around site, steps, inside work, visual checks on panels, reaching, gripping and turning at shoulder height	Decisions about replacement of chemicals, downtime for maintenance, communication with boss	Concentration on panel checks, decision-making, sustained attention, visual perceptual skills	Noise from machinery requiring ear defenders, Outside open to weather and extremes of temperatures Ambient temperature on assessment was 3°C

Steps involved
Check visual panels at 3-hourly intervals
Walk around the site and systematically check all machinery visually and turn valve wheels
Make mental note of maintenance required and record this back in the office
Order new chemicals and parts when needed
Schedule maintenance as required

Specific measurements
Valve wheel at 2 metres from ground. Force on turning not measured. Grip handle diameter of 2 inches
Site is situated on a 1:7 incline. Walks approximately 1 mile each day carrying out these tasks
Metal stairs ranging from 10–20 steps with handrails open to elements
Visual panels at 2 metres, font size at 1.5 cm high.

Figure 2.4 *continued.*

Work study

Work study or work measurement is an engineering concept that is used to address the productivity requirements in industry. It is often used to discover how long it takes to carry out a task and determine performance, to assist in planning production and to establish costs associated with production design and methods. In industrial settings work study engineers may carry out these tasks as part of a work study department. However, a growing number of therapists are now embarking on additional training in these methods to enhance their toolkit to use in vocational rehabilitation. Knowledge of work study can be useful in determining how long it might usually take a person to carry out your client's work, to contribute towards understanding if a client might be able to work at a particular pace and in redesigning the efficiency of activities in a workplace.

A method still widely used is the stopwatch, where cycles of tasks are timed. It is extremely cheap, requires little or no training and is simple. However, using a stopwatch does not account for how much effort a person is putting into their work or how experienced they are; it is also a quite intrusive method for the person being timed. There are many other tools and methods that can be adopted when carrying out work study, but the two that are mentioned here are MODAPTS and MTM. Both of these methods rely not on stopwatch timings of actions performed in a task, but on a 'predetermined motion time system (PMTS)'. PMTS is

'frequently used to set labor rates in industry by quantifying the amount of time required to perform specific tasks . . . requires that the analyst break apart the process into its component actions, assign time values to each action, and sum the times to calculate the total standard time.' Wikipedia (accessed on 20 February 2007)

This is based on the understanding that all human movements take a predetermined amount of time to perform and a considerable amount of research has gone into cataloguing basic work motions. Both methods require extra training and therefore cost money to set up.

Methods Time Measurement

MTM (Methods Time Measurement) (www.mtm.org) was established in 1948 and resulted in common work actions being listed with predetermined times next to them. However, this widely accepted system still requires additional measurements of distances to complete the assessment. Some people say that this makes it quite time consuming to use, but it is very widely used as an accurate measurement and highly respected worldwide (Carey et al. 2001; Zandin Kjell 2003). Several generations of MTM systems have now been developed and training is widely available worldwide. With regards to vocational rehabilitation, MTM is used in some of the standardised functional capacity evaluation tools and can be used to see how closely a person matches the industry standard for performance.

Modular Arrangement for Predetermined Time Standards

MODAPTS (Modular Arrangement for Predetermined Time Standards) (www.modapts.org) is also a predetermined motion time system and is based on empirical studies in the 1960s and 1970s when natural speeds of working were collected. MODAPTS differs from other methods because it focuses on the body part doing the action and not on the distance to be covered or the tool being used. Although work tasks appear to be quite different:

> 'When you look closely, you see that all the work is done by fingers, hands, arm movement, together with eye use and perhaps a little concentration. The differences are that the combinations of the movements and the mental work (i.e. the activities) are different.' (Carey et al. 2001)

The main purpose of MODAPTS to determine the time it takes to do a job when working at an ordinary or standard pace. It cannot, however, account for all the factors that may affect a person's actual working rate, such as environmental considerations, motivation to work, ill-health symptoms.

Health and safety

Health and safety should be a constant consideration when carrying out environment-based assessments related to vocational rehabilitation. As a practitioner carrying out your job, you should be aware of your responsibilities under the Health and Safety at Work Act 1974 (HSW) and the various associated regulations. Under the HSW Act there is a requirement to ensure the health and safety of yourself and others who may be affected by what you do or fail to do. This applies not only to people who have an employer per se but also to self-employed people and workers in the voluntary sector. You should also have awareness of the health and safety obligations that an employer is under detailed in the various regulations. These are the areas that are covered Health and Safety Executive (HSE) (www.hse.gov.uk):

- Risk assessment
- Handling and transporting
- Personal protective equipment (PPE)
- Noise
- Vibration
- Machinery safety
- Ventilation
- Lighting
- Harmful substances
- Safe systems
- Health surveillance
- Selection and training

Before you enter a workplace you need to be aware of any safety requirements, such as personal protective equipment. Going onto a building site will require a hard hat and a high visibility coat, entering a factory may require ear defenders, entering a laboratory may require a white coat, gloves, shoe coverings and goggles. Check the requirements *before* you get to the workplace, otherwise you may not be allowed to carry out your assessment. It is also quite likely that a practitioner will go to a workplace alone to carry out the assessment. So ensure that you are aware of your service's lone working policy and the methods by which you should call for help should you need it. Many services have mobile telephones that employees can take out with them to call for help. Ensure that you have adequate battery life to last your assessment and consider alternatives should your battery fail or you cannot pick up a transmission signal!

Environment-based assessments in the workplace may also have an element of risk assessment based on your client's particular needs. For instance, new risk assessments may be required in a workplace because your client has different needs now compared to when they worked previously. Or clients who now have visual impairments may or may not be at risk of hurting themselves. The hazards will be different and the precautions to minimise the risks may well need to change. The HSE have published advice on risk assessment and recommend the 5-step model:

Step 1: Look for the hazards
Step 2: Decide who might be harmed and how
Step 3: Evaluate the risks and decide whether the existing precautions are adequate or whether more should be done
Step 4: Record your findings
Step 5: Review your assessment and revise it if necessary

If you are not experienced in carrying out risk assessments, you may want to seek the help of an occupational health and safety officer or an occupational health nurse. Both of these professionals have experience in carrying out risk assessments.

Travel to work

As well as considering the environment in which your client will work, it is also helpful to consider how they will get to work and the environments they will encounter during their travelling. Travel to and from work is recognised as a major obstacle in returning to work and one that can sometimes be overcome with some thought and attention to detail. The detail comes from making a thorough assessment relating to each of these areas:

Getting out of the house: Does your client have any difficulties leaving their home i.e. mobility reasons, mental health reasons etc? Are there environmental barriers at home that need addressing?

Travelling distance and time: How far away from the workplace does your client live? How long can it take to get to work? Does this change at different times of the day? What would be the range of times? Does your client have any responsibilities on the way to work i.e. dropping children off at school?

Mode of transport (walking, bus, train, car, aircraft, ferry): What type of transport does your client envisage having to use? What would they find difficult to use? Why? What solution would your client recommend? Does your client have to use several different modes of transport in one journey? What particular problems can this cause?

Cost of travelling: What are the direct costs i.e. petrol, train fare etc? What are the indirect costs i.e. more expensive car, extra time etc? Is your client aware of the cost saving schemes available via HM Customs and Excise, DVLA and the Motability Scheme for car leasing? Is your client aware of the toll concessions that are available to disabled drivers?

Parking at home and at work: What are the parking arrangements for home and work? Can your client access their car easily? How suitable is the pavement, road, driveway, car park for your to access? Does your client have a Blue Badge under the UK's national scheme of parking concessions for disabled drivers organised by the Department for Transport (www.dft.gov.uk)?

Existing support services: Does your client or their employer know about statutory support services such as Access to Work, Mobility Centres, MAVIS etc? Is there practical support from the workplace? Will the workplace allow home working for a period/permanently? Is your client aware of the Disabled Persons Transport Advisory Committee and their role (www.dptac.gov.uk/)?

This is not an exhaustive list and if you reflect on your own travelling to work you may well be able to think of more issues to ask about. Your client may be able to do their job and feel confident about returning to work but unless he or she can actually travel to work, they still cannot move forward. Addressing the issues surrounding travelling to work is of paramount importance to the whole process of return to work.

Summary

Environment-based assessments for work would normally expect to help to identify and describe the demands that a job places on an individual and to evaluate the potential obstacles. The assessments should facilitate you and your client to identify which tasks are likely to be difficult to carry out and why, and to start to consider the solutions. While focusing on the work environment the assessments also touch on physical, functional and psychosocial aspects associated with your client and his or her workplace. Environment-based assessments could include worksite assessments, job analyses, work study, health and safety and travel to work. As well as occurring during sickness absence or unemployment, the assessments could happen while a person is still in work, to help with job retention and to identify if they are having problems and what these problems are.

Considering your role, what makes you the most suitable person to carry out job analyses and worksite visits?

What additional training might you require, where from and how much might it cost?

If you are not the most suitable person, then how will you identify the right person? Where will this person work, who will pay for their services and how much will it cost?

What would a job analysis and a worksite assessment achieve over what your service currently provides?

Chapter 3
ACTION PLANNING

Introduction

This chapter deals with developing action plans. It reflects my own frustrations in attempting to bridge the void between assessment and intervention that often exists in texts talking about rehabilitation. A range of solutions is often given without advice on how to make the right choice for your client. This chapter includes:

- Data analysis
- The obstacles in return to work
- Decision making processes
- Goal setting

A range of assessments have already been identified as potentially useful in helping to identify obstacles that may hinder someone to return to work or to start work for the first time. These assessments have been artificially split into person-based, function-based and environment-based assessments only for the purpose of writing this book. In reality, you would assess your client using a range of assessment tools, concurrently and as appropriate for your client.

It is probably true to say that narrative, i.e. talking and discussing issues with your client will be the main source of information. However, the process does not finish with carrying out an assessment – further work is required to extract meaning from all the information that is gathered. Leach (2002) indicates that in the supported employment model, the first stage to the process is the client-centred analysis of individual strengths and preferences. Often there is an abundance of information and this can make the whole picture rather confusing. Sometimes the cited issue affecting your client, such as back pain or anxiety, may not actually be the barrier to return to work. It is quite common to see a client several times before the real issues start to emerge. It is also common practice to use a cycle of assessment, action planning, intervention and reassessment where the client and practitioner are continuously learning more information and modifying how to achieve the client's goals related to return to work.

Data analysis

Once sufficient data has been collected, it needs to be analysed systematically to interpret and identify the need(s) and ultimately to plan vocational rehabilitation. The analysis should also identify the most appropriate way to facilitate a person during interventions, and answer the question: 'What kinds of supports are going to work best for your clients to reach their goals?'

The analysis is a time for the client and the practitioner to reflect and to assimilate the information that has passed between them. It is a critical time where decisions are made about a person's future, and as such it needs to be taken seriously. If the wrong decisions are taken, your client's working life may be put in jeopardy. All decisions need to be collaboratively made and led by the client and not by other influences such as service targets or the practitioner's own ideas of what is right. Hagedorn (2000) states:

'the individual, the pivot point of the whole endeavour, is an expert in the situation being faced, contributing knowledge, experience and potential, and a desire, however dimly perceived, to make something happen.'

She explains that the client and the practitioner together need to

'understand their situation and embark on the risky journey towards change.'

To effectively organise the information that is gathered, one can turn to one's own professional frameworks and theoretical models as guides.

- In *occupational therapy*, one might choose to use Kielhofner's (1980) model of human occupation
- In *physiotherapy*, one might use the models surrounding musculoskeletal injuries
- In *psychology*, one might use Bandura's (1986) social cognitive theory
- In *vocational rehabilitation*, appropriate models to be mindful of are the supported employment model, the cognitive behavioural psychotherapy model, and Engel's (1977) biopsychosocial model

One might also look to models from other relevant fields such as engineering and business.

The purpose of the models and theories is to give structure and meaning to the situation in which your clients find themselves. They give the practitioner the tools to synthesise the information they gather. As a practitioner, you are accountable for the decisions you make and your clinical reasoning should be evident in your documentation for your own benefit and the benefit of others who may have to take over your caseload and for other people involved with your client, e.g. your interdisciplinary team.

How you set – and the scope of – the goals that you and your client will develop will depend on many variables. The key aspect of the goals is that they will be unique to your client and his or her situation and will reflect the priority of the issues to be addressed in the vocational rehabilitation intervention. Sometimes the planning will be done between just one practitioner and the client. In other situations, the planning will be carried out by a team of different professions, client included (as the expert patient).

How do you currently develop your rehabilitation plans with your clients?

Consider the advice and plans you make. How do you know you are making the right decisions?

Would you know if your plan wasn't working? What would you do to rectify the situation?

Analysing and interpreting data

Analysis and the interpretation of the data that have been collected is an important step in the process of problem solving and rehabilitation planning. If one takes the view that collecting information is important, one should continue this line of action and make use of the data that is now on view. Otherwise, there is little point in gathering data in the first place, other than to create a rapport with your client. I have had many stories told to me by clients who have been in the situation where an hour or more has been spent chatting and giving information to the practitioner only for this information to be unused and inappropriate suggestions and assumptions made – for example, 'Well, as you are a plumber, you definitely won't be able to get back to work with the back ache you have, you should do a computing course.' This has always been conveyed to me as frustrating and demeaning to the client. The next time you see your client for the first time, ask yourself how you are going to use the very valuable and personal information you are about to extract from this individual who is fighting hard to make a difference to their life.

Recording data

It is assumed that the data that has been collected has been documented during collection or very shortly afterwards and that practitioners have followed their own profession or employer's guidelines and best practice on documentation. I use long handwritten notes using a SOAP (Subjective–Objective–Analysis–Plan) format and have done so for many years. Your notes may also be handwritten in paper files or you may work in a paperless system, with all your notes held digitally.

Your individual role as a practitioner will dictate to some extent on how you are able to collect information, the time scales involved and how the analysis and subsequent plans are presented and used. If you are working in a consultative role, you may be asked by an insurance company, an employer or a statutory agency to see an individual who is currently off sick, and to make recommendations for suitable equipment to facilitate a return to work. You may only be able to see the client on one occasion for two hours maximum, while he or she is at home. The information you are able to gather in this situation will be quite different from that of the the practitioner who can repeatedly see the client in different locations and for varying lengths of time. The different situations will derive different sorts of data and different amounts of data and as such you will be more effective in your analysis if you know how you will analyse the data and how you will record this analysis.

Many practitioners, I suspect, are intuitive at this point. They hold a certain amount of tacit knowing in their heads that they then use to problem solve situations, that is the knowledge gained through experiences, shared values and cultural understandings. Knowing how, potentially, to help someone to return to work but not being able to explain it can be both helpful and risky simultaneously. It is obviously time-saving and impressive to the client and an employer to 'know' what the solutions already are, but relying wholly on intuition does not provide the clinical reasoning trail and the documented analysis that is required if more than one practitioner is involved in a client's return to work planning. It is highly unlikely that only one person is involved in this process, unless you are orchestrating your own return to work plan. The analysis may also depend on the instructions from a standardised assessment tool where a specific method will be used to extract meaning from the data or guidance that may be available for non-standardised assessments.

Trustworthy data

Innes and Straker (2002) suggest that by using similar methods as used in qualitative research that one can establish trustworthiness of data. They identified that by including the following areas one could improve the trustworthiness of the data that is collected:

- Audit trail
- Detailed descriptions
- Member checking
- Negative case analysis
- Negotiating recommendations with stakeholders
- Peer debriefing
- Persistent observation
- Ensuring saturation of data
- Structural coherence
- Self-reflection
- Triangulation methods

However, Innes and Straker (2002) also identified that some of these strategies would be more useful in certain work-related assessments than others. They did identify a core of strategies appropriate to all work-related assessments and in relation to data analysis specifically these were self-reflection, peer debriefing and *'frequent analysis of data from various sources and methods through triang-ulation (cross-checking).'*

Grbich (1999) in her book on qualitative research in health warns us that triangulation (gathering information from different points)

'may not serve to consolidate a certain position. It may simply provide more information . . . to deal with.'

As the practitioner gathering the information, you and your client need to decide when sufficient data is gathered to make sense of the situation, to explain what the issues are and to start the process of problem solving, in this case obstacles for return to work.

There are well-used methods to assist with deciphering such information to make some sense of it. In the business world SWOT analyses and mind mapping are two that are used regularly.

SWOT analysis

After a lengthy interview and having scored any standardised assessment, I use a SWOT (Strengths–Weaknesses–Opportunities–Threats) analysis to place all my data on one page and to start to determine where the positive areas and the obstacles sit. An example of a completed SWOT analysis can be seen in Figure 3.1. This SWOT analysis was developed after reflecting on an interview of 2 hours with a client together with the results of two standardised questionnaires and a meeting with the manager at the workplace concerned. The person had been off sick for 6 months following an accident at work and had suffered upper limb injuries requiring surgery.

The SWOT analysis helps to make explicit the client's strengths and weaknesses as well as the opportunities and threats that surround them. The **SW** part usually refers to the individuals themselves, while the **OT** usually refer to external and potential future aspects of a client's situation. However, this is only a tool to help make the analysis of the data easier and is not intended to be a chore or difficult to carry out. So I try not to get hung up on the 'proper' way to use a SWOT analysis.

Mind map

Another technique that can be used to look at analysing a person's situation is developing a mind map.

Mind mapping is a pictorial representation of all the information you and your client have gathered and is said to be a useful way to look at complex issues and to begin to see the interrelationships between issues. A popular psychology writer Tony Buzan developed the idea:

'A Mind Map is a powerful graphic technique which provides a universal key to unlock the potential of the brain. It harnesses the full range of cortical skills

Strengths	Weaknesses
Accident quite recent still looking to resume work	Pain in forearm is constant and makes some tasks impossible
Robust coping strategies being used	Upper limb requiring further surgery
Supportive family	Medical contraindications in place at present
Good self-efficacy for work tasks in spite of disability to upper limb	Some reactions following the traumatic event
No money worries at present	Some anxiety associated with revisiting accident site
Motivated to return to work	
Increasing social contact with peers	Difficulty shifting gears and using handbrake in the car
Independent with all personal care and some household tasks	Unable to perform bi-lateral tasks, carrying, fine co-ordination or fast movements in the affected arm
In spite of pain, able to carry out a range of tasks	
Likes the job and the people at work	Reduced functional independence at home
Recognises the need to return to work as soon as is feasible	Some feelings of abandonment as there has been no contact from the workplace
Questionnaire scores indicate that no formal psychological intervention is required at present	
Opportunities	**Threats**
Workplace offering ongoing training opportunities whilst off sick	Single parent of a young child
	Strenuous parental role at home
Further surgery	No contact from line manager since accident
Further benefit claims may be possible, e.g. Industrial Injuries Benefit	Further surgery may make no difference to functional use of upper limb
Local statutory service may be able to help with transport to work and workstation adaptations	No free rehab available locally looking at return to work specifically
Wide range of adaptations available for desktop computers	Financial worries regarding long-term issues of being disabled
	Worries about being known as disabled
Workplace is willing to look at altering some technologies to reduce keyboard usage	Worried about how to manage being a single parent and cope with the future

Figure 3.1 Example of a completed SWOT analysis.

– *word, image, number, logic, rhythm, colour and spatial awareness – in a single, uniquely powerful manner. In so doing, it gives you the freedom to roam the infinite expanses of your brain. The Mind Map can be applied to every aspect of life where improved learning and clearer thinking will enhance human performance.' (www.buzanworld.com)*

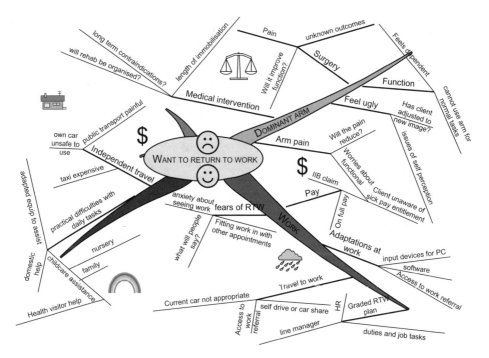

Figure 3.2 Partially completed mind map representing information from assessments and interviews with a client.

Essentially it is a one-page representation of all the information gathered during assessment and interview sessions. Figure 3.2 shows a partially completed mind map of information gathered during a couple of assessments with a client and a workplace. I have used this to start to see if there are any connections between issues that a client may have. If you are able to build a rapport with your client and you are able to spend time together, these pictorial representations can be good to work on collaboratively. They can bring a sense of perspective to you and your client about the issues in hand. The mind map illustrated here has been portrayed using a drawing software package but they are more easily (in my view) drawn by hand.

Problem solving: obstacles in returning to work

One of the main purposes of assessment is to start to understand the predicament in which your client finds him or herself. In vocational rehabilitation, the focus is likely to be on appreciating the situation that is preventing your client from remaining at work or returning to work. The situations you are looking at will undoubtedly include obstacles that are preventing your client from successfully organising their own return to work plan. Through your interpretation and analysis of the data you have collected, you should begin to build a picture to understand your client's situation and of the obstacles (also known as barriers) to returning to work.

Identifying problem areas or issues is realistically done in conjunction with setting goals because it is difficult to identify problems without an endpoint in mind. For instance, most of us could reel off a long list of issues we are not happy about in our lives, but this in itself does not move us forward unless we want to overcome one or a few of the issues. Likewise, if someone has been off work for some time, a lot of time could be spent identifying potential obstacles to return to work without it necessarily being fruitful.

Case study: Hazel

Hazel has been off work with a painful lower back for eight months and she has now lost her job. She is seeing a practitioner through a local statutory service who has carried out some assessments. Hazel listens to the practitioner list all the problems that she has identified during her assessments that are stopping Hazel getting back to her old job. Hazel begins to feel a little deflated. Finally she tells the practitioner that she has no intention of going back to her old job as it involved continuous lifting and carrying and that her goal is to retrain and move into work that requires very little lifting and lightweight carrying only.

The practitioner could have saved an hour or more if she had addressed her client's goals sooner in the process and then looked at the issues relevant to Hazel's goals.

For the purposes of clarity, problem identification and problem solving will be addressed here and goal setting separately.

Business literature and popular texts have addressed the issues surrounding problem identification and problem solving for several decades now. It therefore seems appropriate to be able to borrow some of the tried and tested methods for vocational rehabilitation. Bransford and Stein (1984) developed a model of problem solving based on existing models called IDEAL (a mnemonic for identify, define, explore, act and look) explained in Table 3.1.

Waddell and Aylward (2005) describe the range of potential obstacles in their book, the scientific and conceptual basis of incapacity benefits. They describe obstacles as not being solely within the person or the environment but

> 'commonly result from complex and ill-defined interactions between the individual with a health condition or impairment and their social context, compounded by increasing time and distance from the labour market.'

They go on to explain that obstacles are in part due to the perceptions of the client or individual concerned and the people they are involved with such as their family, co-workers, employer and health professionals.

Waddell and Aylward (2005) have described these multifactorial obstacles and organised them generally as:

Table 3.1 IDEAL problem solving.

Identify	*Actively seek problems that require solutions.* The assessment phase is one way of seeking for issues. Problems will need to be verified and especially those which are complex. In vocational rehabilitation the verification will take place with your client, but potentially with other stakeholders too such as the employer, the GP, family members.
Define	*Represent and define the problem to ensure clarity prior to developing any solutions.* This will usually be carried out collaboratively and the root causes discussed at the same time. It may be helpful to gain other people's points of view as they may well interpret things differently. An insurmountable problem to one person may be seen as easily solved by another because they consider the issues differently.
Explore	*Generate ways of solving the problem,* using creative thinking to develop alternative solutions for consideration. At this stage you might also be addressing your client's problem solving skills and coping strategies. There may be several options open to potentially solve an issue.
Act	*Select the most suitable strategy and put it into action.* Selection may be based on resources available (money, manpower) as well as the will of people to cooperate. The key point here is to act on the chosen strategy, not just plan the strategy.
Look	*Look at how well the solution has solved the problem.* Evaluate it. Re-evaluation of your client should be inherent in your rehabilitation service and as such so should the re-evaluation of the problem-solving strategies. This is a good point at which to carry out self-reflection as a reflective practitioner.

- Personal characteristics
- Psychological factors
- Social factors

Table 3.2 puts some detail into these areas as a way of explaining them further using Waddell and Aylward's (2005) publication, as well as my own experiences.

In the process of developing action plans together with clients, it may be helpful to consider the potential obstacles for return to work under these headings. Indeed while data is being analysed and interpreted, potential barriers to return to work could be explored systematically using these headings as a guide. So we can ask questions such as:

- 'Is there anything in the information that has been gathered to suggest that personal characteristics, psychological factors or social factors are contributing to my client's difficulties in returning to work?'
- 'What factors in my client's personal characteristics and social situation are contributing to obstacles and in what way are they affecting my client's return to work?'

Table 3.2 Multifactorial obstacles in returning to work.

Personal characteristics	Age, gender, family and social background, education, training and skills, work history and work experience	Nearing retirement age
		Time out of work to date
		Family supportive of inactivity
		Marketable work skills
	Physical or mental condition, impairment and functional limitations therein	Fluctuating conditions, medical contraindications
Psychological factors	Personal experience of illness and disability	
	Perceptions and expectations	Of self, others and environments
		Of health and work and sustaining work
	Attitudes and beliefs, emotions, mood, coping strategies	
	Motivation, effort and incentives	Self-efficacy
	Uncertainty	Of own future and the futures of those they are responsible for
Social factors	Culture surrounding health, sickness, disability and work	Popular attitudes to work and health
	Labour market forces	Lack of suitable jobs
		Regional deprivation
	Social and occupational barriers	Access and transport
		Waiting times for healthcare
		Lack of appropriate accommodations and adjustments
	Discrimination, social exclusion	Employer discrimination
		Healthcare professionals' lack of understanding of work related issues
		Bureaucratic criteria to access services unrelated to personal situations
	Financial (dis)incentives	Losing or returning to benefits
		Receiving wages (sick pay entitlement related to return to work)
		Misunderstandings of benefit claims and tax credit systems

Shaw et al. (2002) reported that there are two key constructs that are important in understanding our client's perspective of return to work: the personal meaning of disability and the relevance of return to work. They concluded that:

'Integrating individual perceptions is essential to advancing a multidimensional approach in return to work research.'

It is also fair to say that this can relate to rehabilitation and not just research.

It seems that there is a need during the action planning phase of a vocational rehabilitation programme to educate clients about these research results and concepts. Without our clients also understanding the need to look at the potential obstacles in returning to work (personal characteristics, psychological factors, social factors and individual perceptions of these and the relevance of returning to work) facilitating problem solving could be less effective. Problem solving in this context is referring to the collaborative discovery of the real obstacles for return to work and then the possible ways to mitigate these issues. As mentioned above, the initial reason for being off sick may not actually be the reason that someone remains on sickness absence and it can take some time to establish what might be thought of as the 'real' obstacles. It is suggested here that by using a systematic way, such as the IDEAL method as well as the themes of obstacles to return to work to look at problem solving, one might make better use of one's time and ensure a thoroughness in one's approach to action planning.

Decision making processes

To develop an action plan with a client, one has to make a set of decisions about the information that has been gathered during the assessment phase. As previously intimated, using well-trodden and systematic methods may assist in this process. Many of the decision making methods come from the business world as a result of attempts to ensure that business decisions are made effectively and to help in difficult decision making situations. I would like to suggest that the situation of being off work sick and unable to fathom how to return to work is a difficult situation with difficult choices that need to be made.

The subject of decision making is also the topic of much research in health-related professions as well as in business. There have been many authors and much written about the differences in decision making between experienced and novice practitioners and this topic is often called clinical reasoning (Mattingly 1998; Stephenson 2004; Norman 2005; Unsworth 2005).

'Clinical reasoning is the process used by practitioners to plan, direct, perform and reflect on client care.' Boyt Schell (2003)

Having an understanding of the conceptual basis of clinical reasoning can broaden our skills in this area. In a recent article by Paley et al. (2006) a practical explanation was given regarding a form of clinical reasoning called the In-order-to Analysis. This form of clinical reasoning (written for the occupational therapy literature) suggests that practitioners make decisions based on a client's goal and then work backwards to decide all the intermediate stages and action that is required to fulfill the goal. This analysis of decision making seems sensible and realistic.

Case study: Illustrating in-order-to analysis in clinical reasoning.

James is a double amputee and his practitioner, Simon, has gathered information about James' functioning, his workplace and job and his physical abilities. James wants to return to his old job as a long distance lorry driver in the next six months as he and his wife are expecting their first baby soon and they need a steady income to afford their new child.

Simon suggests that they write down details of James' situation as it is now and the ultimate goal that he wants to achieve. They start with James' goal and consider in what ways his situation will need to change in order to achieve the goal and write these changes down too. They carry on in no particular order but they find that natural sequences of accomplishments need to occur in order to reach James' ultimate goal.

They discover that:

- In order to return to work in his previous capacity a return to work date needs to be established with the employer.
- In order to do this negotiation, a return to work plan needs to be made.
- In order to make a return to work plan James needs to be sure he can get into his lorry and drive it.
- In order for James to drive his lorry, adaptations to James' lorry need to be made and funded for him to drive it.
- In order to make adaptations, a specialist assessment at the heavy goods vehicles assessment centre needs to occur.
- In order for funding to occur, different options need to be explored such as access to work funding, employer funding, insurer funding and so on.

Simon and James go on make shorter term goals based on this exploration of the situation and again break things down further.

Leach (2002) advises us to use all the information that is gathered to assist a client in considering all the viable options and in making appropriate choices. Inevitably there will be some things that need to happen before others and some things that clients will want to achieve before they can even consider the bigger picture. Quite often, the situation that the client finds him or herself in is not easy to navigate around and the priorities are less easy to discern. At times like these, decision making tools may be useful to try out. It is also at these times that your skills as a counsellor (in the word's broadest definition) will come into play. You may need to employ your knowledge of the cognitive behavioural approach to facilitate your client to start to look at their situation and to unravel its complexities.

Deciding on the priorities to set goals with clients is a reflection of client-centred practice and is not the same as considering what the priorities are yourself as the practitioner and then telling the client how to fit in. In the case study, James and Simon decide together what the steps and likely sequence of events should be to reach James' goal. However, Simon might have carried out his assessments and then gone away and developed a plan himself and then presented it to James. James might have accepted the plan, but it still would not have not have been carried out in a truly client-centred manner with full collaboration. Practising in a client-centred manner is one of the tenets of the supported employment model and is also the tenet of many professional groups.

> 'The client-centred approach coupled with an imaginative use of resources (including energy, time and ideas, not just money) will be used to the best effect in resolving areas of difficulty.' (Leach 2002)

Canadian Occupational Performance Measure

The COPM (Canadian Occupational Performance Measure) developed by Law et al. (1998) is a tool that can be used to identify the issues that are important to the client and to develop the priorities as perceived by the client. It is a semi-structured interview to facilitate client-identified problems and collaborative goal setting and

> 'the measure is designed to detect change in a client's self-perception of occupational performance over time.' (www.caot.ca/copm/)

As such it can be used as an outcome measure. Occupational performance in this circumstance covers self-care, productivity and leisure and does not refer to work per se. Clients are asked to identify any activities that they find difficult to carry out and use a 10-point scale to indicate how important these activities are to them. Then the client is asked to choose the five most important problematic activities and asked to rate their performance and satisfaction, again using the 10-point scale (Cohn et al. 2003). Through this process goal setting can occur as well as re-evaluation of goals to monitor changes.

Other tools that may be helpful in the decision making process are those that have emerged from the business world such as the Force Field Analysis and the Urgency Importance Matrix. These two concepts are explained in commonly available decision making publications and ones that you and your client may find helpful in prioritising actions that need or want to be taken to return to working.

Force field analysis

A force field analysis is simply a way of comparing the 'pros' and 'cons' of a particular decision. The representation of a force field analysis was first developed by social psychologist Kurt Lewin. Lewin explained:

> 'An issue is held in balance by the interaction of two opposing sets of forces – those seeking to promote change (driving force) and those attempting to maintain the status quo (restraining forces).' (Value Based Management.net 2006)

Decision or change proposal			
To start to work again as an LGV driver			
Pros	**Value**	**Value**	**Cons**
Need more money for new baby	➡ 6	9 ⬅	No legs to get into cab or to drive with
To boost self-esteem – bored at the moment	➡ 4	7 ⬅	Lost confidence – unsure what I can do
Might lose ranking as a driver if I don't RTW	➡ 7	9 ⬅	Don't have an appropriate vehicle to drive
Family want me to RTW – wife might leave me if I don't RTW	➡ 10	6 ⬅	My employer won't want me back
My insurance payout finishes soon – in 3 months' time	➡ 8	9 ⬅	Cannot see myself driving again
I need to get back to normality	➡ 7	5 ⬅	I don't know how to organise my own RTW
Total	42	45	Total

Figure 3.3 Example of a force field analysis.

Based on information from Mind Tools Ltd (2006), Value Based Management.net (2006) and SkyMark Corporation (2006).

By comparing the positives and the negatives of a decision, one can start to be explicit about them and start to explore the detail and possibly uncover the underlying causes for procrastination (if there is any). It is said that a force field analysis and diagram can be used on many levels including a personal level. Figure 3.3 shows an example of a force field analysis for the broad decision of James to start to work again for an LGV driver. One can use a numeric scale to show the differences or visual elements such as arrows of different sizes, smiley faces or anything that can demonstrate a way of placing value on each of the pros and cons.

The process for developing the force field analysis is to:

1. Describe the situation that faces your client.
2. Describe the situation that they would prefer to be in, i.e. the goal to achieve.
3. Discuss what might happen to the current situation if no action is taken – for example, ask your client: 'What will happen if you don't return to work as an LGV driver?'
4. List all the pros and then all the cons, totalling the scores (determine the values) to each.
5. Discuss the pros and cons to see if they are valid and if they could be altered. For instance, in Figure 3.4 the total scores are fairly similar – is there any

Decision or change proposal			
To start to work again as an LGV driver			
Pros	Value	Value	Cons
Need more money for new baby	→ 6	9 ←	No legs to get into cab or to drive with
To boost self-esteem – bored at the moment. I need to restore some self-worth	→ 7	7 ←	Lost confidence – unsure what I can do
Might lose ranking as a driver if I don't RTW	→ 7	5 ←	Don't have an appropriate vehicle to drive until an adapted one has been located
Family want me to RTW – wife might leave me if I don't RTW	→ 10	6 ←	My employer won't want me back
My insurance payout finishes soon – in 3 months' time	→ 8	4 ←	Cannot see myself driving again unless I have a safe place to practice with hand controls
I need to get back to normality as soon as possible	→ 8	2 ←	I don't know how to organise my own RTW right now, but I could learn
Total	46	33	Total

Figure 3.4 Example of a force field analysis following further discussion.
Based on information from Mind Tools Ltd (2006), Value Based Management.net (2006) and SkyMark Corporation (2006).

positive point that could be strengthened? Is there any negative point that could be weakened? See Figure 3.4 for changes following discussions about the points of pros and cons.

Obviously I have written this force field analysis to emphasise my particular point, and the positives might not always outweigh the negatives so easily. But the idea here is to give your client a visual representation of the values they attach to their situation and to give him or her the chance to explore these issues in a structured manner. By writing their thoughts down on paper, the issues become more explicit to both your client and to you, and decisions about potential goals may come sooner.

Urgency Importance Matrix

Once your client and you have decided on the range of achievements to make, you may need to prioritise them appropriately. The order in which things should

Table 3.3 Urgency Importance Matrix.

Category	Relates to
1. Urgent and important	Crises and meeting deadlines
2. Not urgent but important	Activities that allow you to plan ahead Goal-directed activities
3. Urgent but not important	Activities that often mean responding to other people's demands
4. Not urgent and not important	Activities that make you look like you are busy

After Neenan and Dryden (2002).

be done may be blindingly obvious – such as needing to contact a manager before a client can negotiate a graded return to work plan. However, and quite likely, there will be so many things that could happen concurrently that it is difficult to discern the priorities. The Urgency Importance Matrix is a simple time management technique where you look at what you have to do or want to do and assign them into categories of how urgent and how important you perceive them. This aims to simplify the procedure of deciding on the priority in which to carry out tasks or goals. The technique has been explained fully in Stephen Covey's book *First Things First* (1994) but has also been written about in other texts such as Iain Maitland's book *Managing Your Time* (1999). According to Covey (1994) activities fall into one of four categories (Table 3.3).

Most time should be devoted to activities in category 2 – not urgent but important. Another way of visualising this idea is to put urgent and important on an axis and to plot where different activities/goals should sit. This is illustrated in Figure 3.5.

In Figure 3.5 'having a driving assessment to find correct adaptations' is perceived by the client as both urgent and important; 'practising driving with new controls' is important but not very urgent and 'keeping up to date with relevant paperwork associated with sick leave' is deemed neither urgent nor important, but has to be done (it is routine). This is just another tool that you might find useful when you are in discussions with your client regarding their priorities in relation to their longer-term goal(s). As mentioned previously, writing down on paper what one holds in one's mind makes the thoughts explicit and gives an opportunity to talk about them. You may have a client who is determined to go back to work but who is unsure how to orchestrate the event – discussing what the issues are and the potential goals and then prioritising them allows both your client and you as the practitioner to develop a sound plan. By writing thoughts down on paper in the form of force field diagrams or urgency importance graphs you are developing an audit trail and providing valuable documentation for yourself, your client and your colleagues.

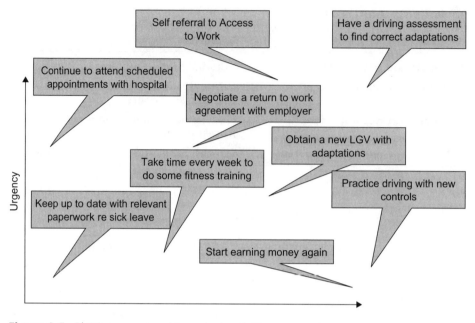

Figure 3.5 Plotting urgent and important activities on an axis.

Goal setting individual programmes

Goal setting is not about picking certain predetermined recipes when your client has a set of particular circumstances. I would suggest that it is a unique plan for your client alone; and as such two clients with persistent back pain and anxiety working on a production line should still have their own unique set of goals. As obvious as this sounds, each client is an individual with unique sets of circumstances. So goal setting needs to be client-led. Setting goals with clients is often mentioned in texts and articles as an activity that is done by the practitioner to the client. But without the full co-operation and involvement of your client in the development of this plan for their life, it can easily move away from ascribing to client-centred practice. While we use our past experiences to be able to better determine the outcomes of our intervention and we can pass this information on to our client, we cannot assume that we know best or are more knowledgeable about our client's situation (although we are likely to have different knowledge that could be helpful in the process of return to work).

Articles sometimes mention goal setting as if we all know how to do it and understand some of the original relevant research. I have always found this part of the whole process of being involved with a client as the most thought provoking and enlightening and often requires tweaking to get the right emphasis on the wording. Leach (2002), when talking about a profile (plan) says it is important to see it as a 'living' document that should take account of individual developments. I agree and echo the need to revisit people's goals with them frequently.

Many professions regularly set goals with their clients and whether they (practitioners and clients) are aware of it or not goal setting is used because it has an effect on motivating people into action. Skinner (2002) says:

'Within the psychological literature, goal setting theory represents one of the most well developed and empirically supported approaches to behaviour change.'

Locke and Latham have spent over 35 years researching the area of goal setting theory in the field of organisational psychology (Locke & Latham 2002). However, their work has emanated out of this particular field and is now used by many different professions and by individuals too making personal life goals. Locke and Latham (2002) state:

'The focus of goal setting theory is on the core properties of an effective goal.'

What is the purpose of goal setting in your service?

How different would your service be without goal setting?

Consider the effects goal setting has on your clients?

Using the theory, goal setting works best when goals are quite difficult to attain, but not so difficult that they cause the client to lose faith in their ability and result in reduced performance. Skinner (2002) explains that results from experiments can show probabilities associated with achieving hard, moderate and easy goals. However, these results are experimental and it is not realistic to work out the probabilities of achieving every goal that a client sets. It therefore comes down to 'best judgement' to set the right challenge. The reasons that goal setting works to change behaviours is said to be because of their influence over:

- The attention and effort towards task relevant behaviours and actions
- The investment of effort and energy in goal-relevant behaviours
- The persistence in striving for goals in the face of obstacles, especially more difficult goals (Locke & Latham 2002; Skinner 2002)

The other aspects that are required for goal success are the basic skills and abilities, commitment to the goals, feedback on individual performance in achieving goals and task complexity. Goal commitment is affected by self-efficacy (Locke & Latham 2002). If your client believes they can achieve the goal and believes they have the strategies to achieve the goal, then self-efficacy will be greater and commitment and persistence to achieve the goal is said to be greater.

Locke and Latham also explain that feedback is required for goals to be effective. This should demonstrate your client's progress in relation to the outcome of the goal and the effectiveness of strategies that are being used to work towards the goal. Feedback on strategies has been shown to be of particular importance in complex tasks. Complex tasks in this context refer to tasks that have several aspects to them, require attention to multiple information cues, and require processing of this information simultaneously with performing challenging physical actions at speed (Skinner 2002). So a complex task might be:

- Writing a letter on a computer every three minutes in a busy and noisy office, while having to answer the telephone each times it rings
- Packing buns into boxes that are coming down an automated line at a particular speed, while checking that the packed boxes are not building up too much, and calling for them to be taken away periodically

Complexity also needs to be seen in context with your client's abilities and needs that you will be familiar with because of the assessments that have been carried out. Some people will be easily able to carry out tasks that you may perceive as complex, so remember not to base the complexity on what you would find challenging or straightforward. Skinner (2002) has two pieces of advice to help with accomplishment of complex tasks:

- Allow time between goal setting and improved performance.
- Allow a period of practice and trial and error in the early stages without the pressure of goal attainment.

Additionally Skinner (2002) and Locke and Latham (2002) advise that short-term goals can be helpful as a stepping-stone to achievement of long-term goals. When one considers this advice, it seems obvious; but short-term goals allow your client to perceive the longer-term goal as more achievable because the distance to it will *seem* shorter. This has an effect on your client's self-efficacy, by increasing your client's belief in their ability to achieve the goal. This will then have a knock-on effect of increasing persistence in attaining the goal because your client believes that they can achieve it.

> Is goal setting an intervention in its own right?
>
> If so, how much of your time should you allocate to it?

Depending on how they are written, these goals can end up being a motivating factor for the practitioner and not the client. Consider how many of us have written or seen written a list of 'goals' that is to all intents and purposes a 'to-do list' for the practitioner? In the context of rehabilitation per se, goals, as I understand, should be written for the client to achieve and not for the practitioner. The acronym SMART has been used for decades now as a guide to writing effective goals. However, there are many descriptions of this acronym now and it may not always be apparent how it should be interpreted. But just as a reminder this is the acronym, as I have always known it. Goals should be written so they are:

S   specific
M   measurable
A   achievable
R   realistic
T   timely

Two newer elements are E and R (SMARTER) to include research pertaining to self-Efficacy and the importance of feedback – Rewards (Rubin 2002).

If you type SMART goals into Google.co.uk you get over 49 million potentially relevant sites! This is obviously a very common topic, and as such I will leave it to those with more space than I have here to discuss. Except to say that I suggest blending the key concepts from goal setting theory and the SMART acronym to write goals effectively.

During an interview and throughout the assessment process you can be asking relevant questions about your client's perceived goals. It may take several sessions before your client has a clear idea of what their goals might look like and they may only be able to consider very short-term goals at first. When talking about return to work specifically, I like to ask my clients some explicit questions:

Do you see yourself working again?'

If the answer is *'no'*: *'What is it you see replacing work?'*

Questioning would not finish here and would continue in a similar vein but asking questions about the preferred activities rather than work.

If the answer is *'yes:'* *'When do you see yourself getting back to work?'*

'How will you know when you are ready to go back to work?'

This question is often difficult for people to answer and I might give them some appropriate examples pertaining to their situation and introducing the idea of monitoring or measuring their performance, for example:

- *'As your work entails you being on your feet for several hours at a time, will you be ready to go back when you can stand and cook a roast dinner and clear up afterwards?'* or
- *'As you are changing your job, do you see yourself being ready when you have explored the job market and tested yourself in interviews?'*

This then leads to the 'in-order-to' questions.

'In order to explore the local job market, what will you need to do first?'

and continue this backward chain as appropriate.

Table 3.4 Action plan template and partially completed goals and action required.

Goals	Action required	By whom	Timescale/ completion date
For James to be able to get in and out of his own lorry cab independently and with good self-efficacy using an adapted seat, if required	To make a referral to the large goods vehicle assessment centre in Wales	James can self-refer	Completed March 2006
	To attend the assessment	James and Simon	Completed April 2006
To be achieved in six months	To write a report and make recommendations for appropriate seating in the cab, listing manufacturers in the UK	Driving centre	Completed May 2006
	To copy report to his employer and Access to Work	James	Due June 2006
	To investigate different manufacturers and obtain accurate costs	Simon and James	By end June 2006
	To liaise with employer about possible funding for vehicle adaptations	Simon and James	By end of July 2006
For James to develop a graded RTW plan with his employer with assistance from Simon	To contact the employer and discuss James' desire to RTW ASAP	Simon	Completed May 2006
For James to feel that the plan is realistic	To arrange a worksite visit and initial meeting with employer	Simon	Completed and scheduled
To be achieved in two months	To attend meeting at scheduled time	Simon and James	Due for June 28th 2006 at 3 pm
	And so on		

Based on previous case study in Figure 3.3.
Template by kind permission of Tim Barnes MA (Cantab) DipCOT, (2006, unpublished)

This is the method that I use and you may have your own tried and tested techniques. Bearing in mind the problem solving and decision making topics that have already been discussed in this chapter, the next stage would be to bring all this information together into an 'action plan'. Table 3.4 is an example of an action plan template. The action plan has been written based on Hazel's case study on page 85. The goals in vocational rehabilitation are as wide and varied as the clients that you see, some being directly related to work and returning to work and some seemingly less relevant but are nevertheless a pathway that may lead your client to working again or remaining in work.

In this example, if a SMARTER goal was written, then a separate column detailing the types of feedback (the **R** part of the acronym) may need to be added or the practitioner in could detail this information. You may want to have a separate column that states the outcome that is actually achieved, or the start and finish dates and a comments column (Leach 2002). From my own experience I have found that the simpler the form is to complete, the less time it takes and therefore the more likely I am to continue completing it.

If your client is being seen by a single discipline as part of their vocational rehabilitation, then one might presume that the two individuals involved would carry out the goal setting. If your client is attending a service for vocational rehabilitation then presumably the goal setting will occur between the client and either several members of the team or a specific person working as an intermediary between the team and the client. It will depend on the type of team you work in and the way in which you communicate with each other. If you work in an interdisciplinary team where you all share a certain amount of your skills and knowledge, then your client's action plan may reflect this with one person carrying out several different roles or several people carrying out similar roles. If you work in a multidisciplinary team, each of you may have your own particular roles to carry out in relation to your client's action plan. As long as you and your client understand what is going on and the action plan is being carried out, monitored and changed to match your client's changing needs, then that seems appropriate.

It may be that your client has several action plans or just goals to achieve through attending several different services. Who owns that action plan? It seems simple to say, but it is the client who owns them, not a service. However, in a fragmented system of health and social care, it is often difficult for there to be one action plan or one set of goals that everyone will sign up to as being appropriate for the client. This is obviously a problem with how vocational rehabilitation services are set up and not a problem with the client's action plan per se. Your client needs to feel empowered to take his or her action plan with them to different services and to be confident enough to say that other services need to fit in with their goals. If you have the opportunity to advocate for your client then do so.

What happens to your client's goal sheet or action plan when they are referred on to additional services that refuse to communicate with you?

How do you manage this sort of situation? The action plan is not a static piece of documentation and as such it requires regular monitoring and updating to review progress that is made by your client. In your review meeting you need to consider what it is you are going to review as well as how this information will be gathered and these elements may need to be put into the design of an action plan document:

- What is important for your client to have feedback about?
  - Distances from reaching goals
  - Methods on achieving goals
  - Support that is being offered
- What does your service require feedback about?
  - Costs to date
  - Outcome measures
  - Number of hours rehabilitation utilised
  - Miles travelled
  - Staff numbers utilised
  - Grades of staff utilised
- What do the team members (practitioners) require feedback about?
  - Timeliness of interventions
  - How well appointments were organised
  - Communication skills
  - How well rehabilitation worked
  - The appropriateness of interventions

Summary

In Chapter 3 we looked at action planning – the activities that can be carried out after assessment (usually) and before the vocational rehabilitation starts. Issues around analysing data, developing an understanding of the obstacles in return to work, the processes that can be used in decision making and goal setting have all been included in this chapter. When you are planning rehabilitation with your client, who is essentially being persuaded to change the way they currently function to move to a different status quo, it seems pertinent to look at methods to facilitate this change so it occurs in a positive way. How you use action planning, the types of goals you are realistically able to set and how often you review the action plan will on the whole depend on the service in which you work and your own professional background. A client-centred approach has been highlighted as the most appropriate for engaging someone in vocational rehabilitation, and regardless of service restrictions or your own points of view, your client should be the focus during the action planning process.

Chapter 4
INTERVENTIONS

Introduction

In Chapter 3 we looked at developing action plans through problem-solving methods and goal identification. In many ways, action planning is the simpler part of vocational rehabilitation, but it is meaningless on the whole unless the plan is implemented. Once the action plan has been developed, it should continue to guide the vocational rehabilitation interventions, receiving the same amount of attention and energy that was used in its development. The goals should be framed in time and these will act as target dates and points at which to recheck the action plan and modify it as required. The action plan is not the entirety of the vocational rehabilitation programme – support in achieving the goals is required and it is the careful choice of interventions that will provide the support to achieve the goals.

When people engage with rehabilitation, there is a perception that something is being done to them to remedy a particular problem or issue. When vocational rehabilitation is mentioned, it is interesting to consider what is actually meant by this term. To some people it could mean help with returning to a job, to others it could mean training to obtain a job, to others it doesn't relate to jobs at all but to meaningful occupation, voluntary work or engagement in activity that is purposeful. But both rehabilitation and vocational rehabilitation probably still conjure up ideas of having something done to you. Semantics are less of an issue when you describe what you do with your client and there is an argument to use different phrases to describe different interventions with people rather than lumping them all together as vocational rehabilitation or work rehabilitation.

These days rehabilitation is about a journey that a client takes, along which several practitioners (of which some might be termed professionals) help with the navigation. It is about learning to understand the client's goals related to the broad topic of work and as a practitioner, helping your client to find ways to accomplish the goals, giving them feedback about their performance and strategies and finishing the intervention at the right time. This is what William Beveridge said in 1942 when describing rehabilitation:

> *'Rehabilitation is a continuous process by which disabled persons should be transferred from the state of being incapable under full medical care to the state of being producers and earners.' (Social Insurance and Allied Services, HMSO 1942)*

Interventions that look at the goals associated with work are as broad as they are long and that is the whole point really. Each client is an individual and as such has unique goals that they want to achieve and therefore each individual requires unique methods for goal attainment. However, Waddell et al. (2004) say:

> 'There is considerable uncertainty about what "rehabilitation" is, and about its (cost) effectiveness, particularly for the common health problems that cause most long-term disability and incapacity.'

Perhaps it is the individuality of rehabilitation that makes it challenging for some people and organisations to grasp and more challenging in research terms to elicit firm evidence. Or perhaps current rehabilitation is not designed for the common health problems that dominate sickness absence, being designed instead for the complex severe medical condition. Waddell et al. (2004) say:

> 'Rehabilitation must focus instead on identifying and overcoming the health, personal/psychological, and social/occupational obstacles to recovery and (return to) work.'

In this chapter we will first look at the general considerations surrounding vocational rehabilitation, then look at the interventions that might be offered associated with health and social care, then look at workplace interventions, then work rehabilitation and finally career choice and career decision making.

General considerations

This chapter shows which systems are currently organised in the UK. The way we generally make our connections and referrals is by considering the various systems such as the healthcare system and then considering the sectors within that, such as the voluntary sector. I want to move from looking at interventions for particular diagnostic groups such as cardiac conditions or mental health conditions and instead focus on **all** relevant interventions that might help someone returning to work, looking for work or making a career choice.

Whether an employer pays for the work that is done, or the payment is purely in terms of self-satisfaction, is somewhat immaterial. If someone is attending a specific environment to carry out meaningful occupations then there will be similar (not identical) issues. There will be issues related to the environment, issues related to the tasks and issues related to the person to address. If your client is self-employed, they will have similar issues about productivity that a small employer might have. If your client is doing voluntary work, they will have similar issues of health and safety in doing a particular task as will people working in a large factory. If you have clients with common mental health problems and you also see clients with physical problems, their issues about returning to work are likely to be similar – worries about the future, worries about what people at work will say, worries about what happens if they go off sick again. The issues will not be identical, but the broad worries will be similar because you are dealing with work and how human beings function.

Obstacles in return to work and rehabilitation

Obstacles in returning to work have been mentioned throughout this book and it is pertinent to mention them again. Vocational rehabilitation should focus on those barriers and obstacles to work, which also commonly include issues that might traditionally be considered outside of the work topic such as wellness, childcare issues, or financial concerns. Under the biopsychosocial model, it is important to consider all areas of a person's life when talking about working and returning to work. To appreciate the obstacles that disabled people meet in everyday life, including return to work, one needs to understand the social model of disability. In doing so, one begins to appreciate the exclusion and discrimination that disabled people live with and the barriers that are raised to prevent their full participation in society (TUC 2006b).

Traditionally, the medical model has been used for all aspects of people's lives when they have an impairment. It looks primarily at disease and the impairment and measures to ameliorate the situation or ways to cope with the impairment. However, Waddell and Aylward (2005) have explained that there is limited correlation between symptoms, impairment and disability. It seems logical to assume that only focusing on impairments and attempting to remedy them will not necessarily lead to improved functioning and participation in society (which would include work if appropriate). This does not mean that the medical model is futile. In an acute medical emergency it serves to alleviate suffering, disease and dying, which is what any of us need if we are acutely unwell. But this model does not translate easily into the venue of rehabilitation, where individuals require less of a biological emphasis and more of social emphasis that helps them to re-engage in society (and work if appropriate). The models and approaches that aim for participation in society seem to be the most appropriate. The World Health Organization's 2002 International Classification of Functioning, Disability and Health (ICF) is a classification of health and health-related domains that describe body functions and structures, activities and participation. The domains are classified from body, individual and societal perspectives. Since an individual's functioning and disability occurs in a context, ICF also includes a list of environmental factors. The social model and the ICF act as frameworks by which vocational rehabilitation practitioners can frame their vocational rehabilitation programmes, not necessarily the content per se but the overall design and tenets.

Some of the most important obstacles in returning to work come from beliefs that we hold and the interpretations we have about ourselves in our world. Hansen et al. (2004) looked at factors that are significant for return to work early on in a person's sick leave. They found that it is the impact of many factors that has influence on return to work and that the strongest predictive factor

'concerned the individual's expectations concerning the likelihood that they would return to work.'

Shaw et al. (2002) found two key constructs in attempting to understand return to work from the perspective of the individual. These constructs were the personal meaning of disability and return to work relevancy. In helping someone to return to work, Shaw et al. (2002) ask us to listen to a person's own perspectives of their impairments and the relevance that work has. In doing so, appropriate vocational rehabilitation can be designed to reflect the individuality of the client. Hansen et al. (2004) advise rehabilitation professionals to use this kind of information

'to consider the people's attitudes and their resources for adaptation'

and not to use the information to exclude someone from potential interventions. The researchers found that there were several parts to the two key constructs.

- The meaning of disability
  - The illness experience
  - The impact of disability on individual needs
  - The process of getting better
- Return to work relevancy
  - The meaning of work
  - Personal motivations for working
  - Opportunities and expectations of work and the workplace

There is therefore, great merit in ensuring that the meaning of disability and return to work relevancy are parts of the vocational rehabilitation programme – to help individuals explore these constructs and to help individuals understand what their vocational rehabilitation programme would look like for them.

How does your service approach the individuality of each client?

Does your service fit your client or does your client have to fit in with your service?

Rehabilitation services

Another of the obstacles to return to work must be the availability of local resources and services, competent and trained staff and workable referral pathways. These could be viewed as societal or systemic – in that the barriers lie within the existing systems of health and social care. The TUC in 2000, in *Getting Better at Getting Back* said:

'There needs to be adequate provision of high quality rehabilitation services, and access to them.'

However, there is a recognition that while there are many providers of vocational rehabilitation in the UK, the services are patchy and are often designed to meet the needs of particular groups rather than to serve the wider population.

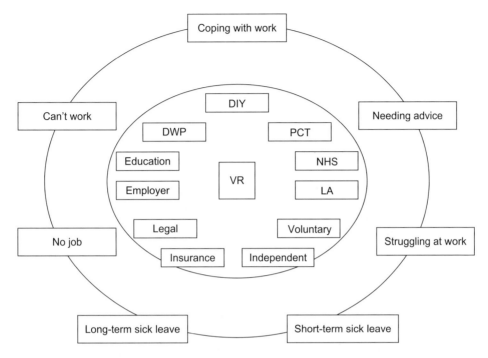

Figure 4.1 Vocational rehabilitation, the sectors it can sit in and the stages at which vocational rehabilitation may be required.

Ideally the NHS would be the provider for health-based vocational rehabilitation – as they did in 'the good old days'. But vocational rehabilitation is not just related to health – it covers areas of social care, education and careers and employment, so it does not naturally sit in any one domain (Figure 4.1).

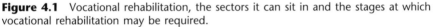

Who would you choose to be in your vocational rehabilitation service in terms of professional representation, experts but not necessarily professional and service user involvement?

Consider why you have made your particular choices. Have you covered all the elements that your clients require?

Now ask your clients who else you need.

One of the issues facing commissioners of vocational rehabilitation is that of staff competency and assured service quality. Debra Perry from the International Labor Office says:

'Quality programs must be assured so that people with disabilities can compete in the workplace. People with disabilities and employers require quality, *responsive services. Methods for ensuring quality include developing skills and competencies among vocational rehabilitation personnel, instituting management information and quality control systems, assuming a multisectoral approach to providing services, conducting follow-up and outcomes studies, administering and analyzing customer satisfaction surveys, and exploiting the use of technology.' (Perry 2001)*

While vocational rehabilitation services remain unregulated, anyone can claim to be an 'expert' in helping people to return to work. But how is this measured, and who determines the definition of a competent vocational rehabilitation consultant or practitioner? Some examples of contemporary work in this area are:

- The *Vocational Rehabilitation Association* (VRA) published a consultation paper called *The Way Forward: recognising and accrediting education and training provision for the vocational rehabilitation professional* (VRA 2006). This paper was a result of work by a task group set up by VRA to examine the development of education and training in the vocational rehabilitation profession. (www.vocationalrehabilitationassociation.org.uk)
- The *College of Occupational Therapists* is developing a position statement on vocational rehabilitation. (www.cot.org.uk)
- The *Faculty of Occupational Medicine* is developing a framework for occupational medicine education in medical schools. (www.facoccmed.ac.uk)
- The *Association of British Insurers* develop ideas on competencies for vocational rehabilitation practitioners and services in its document *Care and Good Health: Improving Health in the Workplace* (2006). (www.abi.org.uk)

We will need to wait and see how these new initiatives develop in the UK. In five to ten years' time, the societal or systemic barriers to return to work may be reduced by the widespread introduction of modern rehabilitation services that are staffed by competent practitioners providing quality measured services. The TUC (2006b) says:

'Monitoring and scrutiny of providers is also an important part of the task of maintaining standards.'

This may well require the mobilisation of new services and the extending of existing services:

- In the field of education within universities, colleges and other educational providers to educate practitioners to a certain standard.
- In the development of an appropriate regulatory body for the practitioners and the services themselves.
- In current health and social care services, extending existing rehabilitation services to always include vocational rehabilitation, and to build new (vocational) rehabilitation services where none exist.

- As the new welfare reforms start, many more vocational rehabilitation services will be required at a local level to meet the increased demands of services to help in the rolling out of Pathways to Work and the Condition Management Services to all areas in the UK, not just the current pilot areas.
- Within the employer sector, to support employers through the vocational rehabilitation pathways, which may involve extending current occupational health services to include occupational (vocational) rehabilitation services available to all employers and those who are self-employed.
- Within the insurance sector, to facilitate rehabilitation on all policies by all insurance providers, providing incentives to employers and individuals for reduced sickness absence and higher return to work rates.

Waddell and Aylward (2005) talk of modern concepts of rehabilitation that relate to the

'Council of Europe (1996) recommendations on a coherent and global policy for the rehabilitation of people who are disabled or who are at risk of becoming so.'

They describe modern concepts of rehabilitation as lifting

'the goal from a pessimistic accommodation of limitations to more optimistic restoration of full and normal work.'

Waddell and Aylward's modern rehabilitation would involve:

- Principles being integrated into clinical management and occupational management
- Addressing and overcoming health-related, personal and social/occupational barriers to recovery and return to work
- Restoring normal activity levels and participation
- Returning to full and normal work
- Condition management principles
- Employment support measures
- Services that are designed and appropriate for common health problems

(Waddell & Aylward 2005)

If we agree with Waddell and Aylward in their idea of modern vocational rehabilitation, then what skills are required in the workforce to supply these contemporary services? The NHS Knowledge and Skills Framework may be able to provide a structure by which to assess an individual's competence in vocational rehabilitation. Burbidge (2003) suggests that if there are to be improvements in the accuracy and specificity of the predicted response to rehabilitation, outcomes need to be measured in a more meaningful way. This may then correct the mismatch between the practitioner's goals and the client's goals and provide interventions to fit the client instead of choosing clients to fit the interventions.

Referral pathways

How do clients access vocational rehabilitation services and who makes the referral? A sensible way of approaching this is to consider the person who is working, the person who is on early sick leave, the person who is on longer-term sick leave and the person who no longer has a job.

If someone is already working but needs some advice about a mild pain or ailment, they usually have to identify the right source of information themselves.

- They might source self-help material from their GP surgery or library, or from the Internet.
- The workplace or an insurance policy may have a telephone counselling/advice service.
- If someone is already working but is struggling, they usually have to investigate the source of potential help.
- They might approach their GP for advice and referral on to an appropriate health professional (if it is a health-related condition that is causing the difficulty).
- They might approach the employer's occupational health department for advice or referral on for relevant health-related interventions. An enlightened employer may have workplace-based drop-in sessions with rehabilitation professionals where employees can ask advice and receive help/rehabilitation.
- For a social problem, they might approach an alternative source such as the housing department or welfare rights advisor.
- They might refer themselves to the Access to Work service at Jobcentre Plus to see if workplace adjustments could make their working life easier.

If someone takes sick leave for seven days or more, they would normally see their GP to obtain a sickness certification. At this point:

- The GP may not offer any help, and the individual might have to ask their GP for advice about return to work and referral on to an appropriate health professional.
- The GP may offer advice about the long-term effects of sickness absence and appropriate local rehabilitation services and other social services such as welfare rights. The GP may refer the individual on to traditional health services and then the primary or secondary health provider may refer or provide vocational rehabilitation as a service.
- The GP may suggest the person sees an advisor in the surgery (if this service exists) who can advise them about the long-term effects of sickness absence and give advice about appropriate local services that may be able to help with return to work per se, or related obstacles to return to work.
- The GP may suggest that the individual refers him or herself to the disability services team at Jobcentre Plus for advice about return to work. They may be able to advise and help with workplace adjustments (through Access to Work) and looking at alternative work (disability employment advisor).
- The employer may contact the individual via the line manager, human resources or occupational health, depending on the individual policies, and

discuss ways of assisting the individual to return to work. Or the employee may contact the workplace for advice.

Until the person reaches 26 weeks on sick leave, the GP should regularly see the individual and continue to give appropriate advice and make referrals to appropriate local services. The workplace should also maintain regular contact with the person on sick leave and continue to look at ways in which to facilitate the return to work of their employee. Once a claim has been made for benefits, new opportunities are opened to them through services funded by the Department of Work and Pensions (DWP). In broad terms these services are designed at this stage to look at workplace adjustments, preparing for return to work and to managing the health condition. At the 26-week mark, the GP should still be involved in signing sickness certificates and therefore still involved in actively encouraging and facilitating their patient back to work. Therefore the employee, the GP, the employer and now Jobcentre Plus are both involved in this pursuit.

If your client no longer has a job to return to, they may still be able to access services from Jobcentre Plus and other services funded by DWP that may be delivered by different providers at a local level. The personal advisor at the Jobcentre may be able to refer the individual through to local services that are funded by DWP such as work preparation projects or Workstep; or through to job brokers and career advice services. Local health charities may be able to provide some support in returning to work and social enterprise schemes may also be able to help. Your client may be involved in NHS services at a primary or secondary level, and these services may provide vocational rehabilitation services and integrate with other non-NHS vocational rehabilitation services locally and nationally.

However, it is likely to become more complicated to navigate all the possible local opportunities simply because no one service has information about all of them. As yet, there is no standard mapped-out way to access vocational rehabilitation in the UK. Currently at any point of someone working or wanting to work, they need to know which sector or system they have to access to receive the right kind of vocational rehabilitation (help to return to work). They then have to rely on the person in that sector – e.g. the GP in the local primary care trust (PCT) – having the right information about the appropriate local services to refer the individual, such as the disability employment advisor, condition management programme, or the local occupational therapy department. Referral mechanisms are ad hoc and patchy.

Vocational rehabilitation is not a profession in its own right in the UK and this may be adding to the difficulties with accessing appropriate return to work services. Vocational rehabilitation is very broad and can sit under many sectors, as seen in Figure 4.1.

In 2004 the Association of British Insurers (ABI) (www.abi.org.uk) published a research paper, *Availability of Rehabilitation in the UK*. They commissioned this piece of work because they recognised that the demand for rehabilitation services and vocational rehabilitation services was on the increase due to major changes in government policy. The document explains:

'The Employment National Training Organisation (ENTO) completed an occupational mapping exercise, reported in 2002, that identified that there was a 'core' group of some 9000 to 10 000 practitioners in the UK who could be said to be spending all, or a substantial part of, their time working with disabled people to help them secure or retain employment. In addition, there is a far larger 'non-core' group of some 700 000 who assist with the employment or retention of disabled people.' (Wright et al. 2004)

ENTO proposed the following clusters of core occupations, which are broader than the sectors mentioned in this book (Wright et al. 2004):

- Medical and healthcare, e.g. occupational therapy, physiotherapy
- Work preparation, e.g. job coaching, work assessment, careers guidance
- Placement and brokerage, e.g. advocacy, job matching
- Workplace access, e.g. job analysis, access mediation
- Workplace integration and retention, e.g. technology adjustments, workplace induction support

Your client may need to dip into vocational rehabilitation services at different times during their life and Figure 4.1 illustrates the proliferation of sectors that need to be navigated to get to the vocational rehabilitation services locally. Table 4.1 explains these sectors in a little more detail.

Table 4.1 The sectors associated with provision of vocational rehabilitation services.

Sector	Relevance to vocational rehabilitation
Do it yourself (DIY)	The individual/employee organises their own vocational rehabilitation by reorganising their workload, workspace, paying for their own physiotherapy, counselling etc. People who are self-employed or those who are very motivated to work might do this.
Primary care trust (PCT)	The GP and other surgery staff may provide advice and signposting to local services. The GP may refer on for health-related rehabilitation and necessary medical interventions.
The NHS (mostly secondary care)	The hospital occupational therapy and physiotherapy departments may provide some rehabilitation. They may also be able to signpost to other appropriate local services. Local Expert Patient programmes will be able to provide support and signposting for specific diagnostic groups.
Local authority (LA)	The Occupational Therapy departments may be able to pursue work issues with their clients. Support workers will also have a large role in facilitating their clients in work, if this is appropriate for their client. Some councils now have a return to work programme to recruit people into council vacancies and to then support people during their employment. There are referral criteria and some projects are time limited. Disability champions are emerging throughout councils and they may be able to provide support and advice to other council employees.

Table 4.1 *continued.*

Sector	Relevance to vocational rehabilitation
Voluntary organisations	There may well be charities and volunteers who provide services to support people into work. The CVS (Centre for Voluntary Services) may well have a list. Organisations will be funded through governmental and non-governmental initiatives and will have different referral criteria. They may provide job brokering, work preparation, supported employment, job placements and so on. Most are fairly small and may have experienced staff on board.
Private companies	Case management and rehabilitation companies are emerging in the UK and there may be a local provider. They will have specific referral criteria and will usually require payment for services. These companies are used by the legal and insurance sectors.
Insurance providers	Insurers may have provision for rehabilitation and vocational rehabilitation as a benefit to a particular policy. When an individual or an employer makes a claim on a policy, this will initiate the rehabilitation. They may employ their own rehabilitation staff to provide the services or outsource this service to a private company and sometimes a voluntary sector project or the NHS.
Legal sector	Solicitors may commission rehabilitation for their client who is pursuing litigation for an accident that may have happened at work or in another location, i.e. car accident. The solicitors may organise the rehabilitation or they may have an in-house case manager who can do this for them. The rehabilitation services may be from a variety of settings as with the insurance providers.
Employers	Depending on the policies of the particular employer, occupational health services may be used, and a 'works doctor' who may or may not have occupational health training may be employed to provide assessment and advice. Local trades unions representatives may be able to support a member who is off sick. Vocational rehabilitation in the form of workplace adjustments, education to employers and employees, referral on to other external rehabilitation services may all be part of the services on offer.
Education sector	This has been included because so many students who attend colleges and universities are in part-time work, training for a particular job or intending to go on to work. The student support office may have a disability officer who is able to organise adjustments to assist the student to access the course materials and buildings. This is based on the same tenet as vocational rehabilitation. If the experience is positive at college, the students may learn how to help themselves and go on to a positive work experience.
Department of Work and Pensions (DWP)	There are many pilots and short-term projects that DWP are running throughout the UK and these change. The Disability Services Team helps disabled people in returning to work. Personal Advisors assist people claiming benefits to access relevant Jobcentre Plus and DWP-funded programmes locally. The Pathways to Work programme is due to be rolled out through out the UK (including the Condition Management element) and this will be available to everyone on the current Incapacity Benefit and the proposed Employment and Support Allowance (ESA).

If vocational rehabilitation includes stakeholders from many different sectors, these stakeholders must be aware of this fact and must support the rehabilitation process and not hinder it.

'Sickness absence and return to work are social processes that depend on work-related factors and employer attitudes, process and practice.' (Waddell et al. 2004)

The TUC report *Jobs for Disabled People* (2006b) explains that thousands of people are injured at work each year in the UK, but so few employers have proper rehabilitation policies in place that many employees never return to work. In January 2006, the Chartered Institute of Personnel and Development (CIPD) (www.cipd.co.uk) published a survey it had carried out with 750 employers in the UK. It was a stark reminder of the attitudes some employers hold about those people with a long-term history of sickness absence and incapacity. The survey showed that one employer in three would deliberately exclude people with long-term sickness histories during recruitment.

It is not just the responsibility of the employer. Health providers also have a responsibility to be aware that they are stakeholders and they need to provide adequate resources to help patients return to work. This might be in the form of hospital or community rehabilitation, consultancy services, signposting, etc. Following its report *Monitoring Poverty and Social Exclusion* (2005), the Joseph Rowntree Foundation is encouraging all health and rehabilitation professionals to make their disabled clients aware of schemes to help them to return to work. They say an estimated 800 000 disabled people are actively seeking work but are unable to secure a job. Work as such is not only one of the goals: work is generally therapeutic in itself and therefore an essential part of rehabilitation.

'Every health professional who treats patients with common health problems should be interested in and take responsibility for rehabilitation and occupational outcomes. That requires radical change in NHS and health professionals' thinking.' (Waddell et al. 2004)

The TUC (2006b) and the Disability Employment Coalition (2004) urged the Government to resource and publicise the relevant departments within DWP such as Access to Work. The Disability Employment Coalition (2004) said in its report that 74% of employers had not heard of Access to Work. When one considers all the potential barriers to returning to work, one can begin to understand the responsibility that should be held in different sectors. The TUC identifies barriers inside and outside the workplace, including such as housing, education and transport

'which make it difficult for many disabled people to compete on equal terms in the labour market.'

The Disability Rights Force has recommended that employment tribunals when conducting discrimination cases under the Disability Discrimination Act have similar powers as those of the Employment Rights Act. This would upgrade the recommendation for re-engagement to ordering the re-engagement (TUC 2006b).

The individual who is engaging in the process of return to work also has some responsibilities.

'Rehabilitation is an active process that depends on the participation, motivation and effort of the individual, supported by health care and employers.' (Waddell et al. 2004)

We can begin to see the importance of every stakeholder being aware how their services, policies and procedures affect people returning to or entering work and how responsibility must be shouldered by all these sectors effectively to help people to return to work.

Implementation of vocational rehabilitation

There are possibly two main models of implementation used in vocational rehabilitation in the UK. Other frameworks and models are also useful, but these two in particular are strongly influencing vocational rehabilitation interventions at present.

- *Case management* is a way of managing clients' rehabilitation without necessarily performing the interventions oneself.
- *Supported employment* is a way of helping people into sustainable open employment.

They are not mutually exclusive and so could in theory work together in a service. Government departments are advocating both strategies and both have track records now with case management being first coined in the USA in the 1960s and supported employment also developed in the USA in the 1970s and 80s.

Case management model
In the UK there are two case management organisations:

- BABICM (British Association of Brain Injury Case Managers) (www.babicm.org)
- CMSUK (the Case Management Society of the UK) (www.cmsuk.org)

The definition of case management is:

'A collaborative process which assesses, plans, implements, coordinates, monitors and evaluates the options and services required to meet an individual's health care, educational and employment needs, using communication and available resources to promote quality, cost effective outcomes.' (CMSUK)

Case managers in the UK hold a professional qualification and are registered and regulated by their own professional body such as the Health Professions Council, British Association of Social Workers and the Nursing and Midwifery Council. There are standards of practice that have been developed for case managers in the UK and postgraduate education is also now available specifically directed at case management.

Case management is not only used for vocational rehabilitation – in fact, when it was first developed in the USA it was to manage complex and difficult cases. Case management is a particularly useful approach to use when managing someone whose rehabilitation and re-engagement into society falls between several different boundaries and professional groups. The concept of a key worker has been used for decades in the UK and case management takes this some steps forward by being the first point of contact for a client and the wide array of people and services from different sectors that might be involved. Those professions who have traditionally liaised between many sectors to organise housing, discharge planning, equipment and adaptations for clients find it easy to fit into the role of a case manager.

The case manager would normally be assigned to a client as early on as possible and the manner in which this occurs will depend on the referring agency and the service for which case management is being provided. A case manager assesses their client and in terms of vocational rehabilitation would be identifying the barriers to work amongst other issues such as financial issues, independence in daily activities and most of the assessment areas that have been mentioned in Chapter 2.

Essential elements to case management are:

- Building a rapport with the client
- Developing the action plan with the client
- Planning co-ordination, which could include detailed costs for all the proposed parts of the action plan

The case manager would not normally be expected to provide treatment her or himself. Some organisations will have case managers who only maintain telephone contact with their client following the initial assessment, with all the face-to-face work being done by vocational rehabilitation specialists. In other organisations such as an interdisciplinary team, the case manager may also be a nurse or an occupational therapist whose intervention skills need to be used actively for a service to survive. The role of the case manager is to support the client through his or her vocational rehabilitation and to act as an advocate on their behalf when required. Although not necessarily providing hands-on treatment, the case manager would have a role in organising adaptations to environments and equipment, negotiating with employers, personal advisors at Jobcentre Plus, solicitors and insurers about return to work planning and referring for welfare rights advice and health interventions (and this list is not exhaustive).

If a decision is taken by one service that affects the overall plan negatively, the case manager's role is to attempt to rectify the problem. For instance, if someone's housing benefit was stopped and this caused immediate financial difficulties, the case manager might call the housing department and discuss the matter (with prior permission) and establish how to rectify the financial worry the client was left with. In reality there may be a plethora of ways to intervene in a situation like this. The important management issue is that money worries are a real concern for people and can be the biggest barrier to work – so it is very important to deal with them as soon as possible.

Supported employment model

In the UK the association dedicated to supported employment providers is the British Association for Supported Employment (BASE) (www.afse.org.uk), which currently represents over 200 agencies throughout the UK. The aims of BASE are to:

- Assist people with disabilities by encouraging the provision of support into employment.
- Endorse and promote quality standards in the delivery of Supported Employment.
- Nurture and encourage the setting up of new supported employment services.
- Promote the training of supported employment personnel throughout the UK.
- Provide a regular, detailed information, advisory and development service to association members.
- To liaise and negotiate with national and international government and non-government organisations to promote the aims of the Association. (www.afse.org.uk)

The role of supported employment is to:

'Arrange supports for the individual with disabilities in such a way as to promote a long-term employment experience without the need for continued outside support and intervention from a human service source.' (Callahan & Garner 1997 in Leach 2002)

There are understood to be principles underpinning supported employment and Leach (2002) describes these as:

Self-determination: to be proactive in making choices about all aspects of your life, even the choices that lead to miscues and have to be renegotiated.

Person-centred planning (PCP): a process of discovery of individual aims, aspirations and skills that focuses on the individual rather than service provision constraints, a collaborative effort by the individual and those willing to commit time and energy to support the individual in achieving goals.

Social and economic inclusion: regular life experiences that include family, friends, acquaintances, a job and a social life.

Choice: having the support, advice and information to make real choices and the support to be able to follow through and make those choices a reality.

Employable: all individuals who want to work can work in a job that matches their skills and needs.

Work: people learn about life by living. Everyone learns about work in work, making mistakes, making friends and developing skills in real work situations.

Individual placement is the favoured approach these days where the job that the client is being introduced to is *not* owned by the service provider. A job coach will commence the employment phase with intensive training in the workplace, engaging a work colleague to eventually support the client when it is required. This helps to make the placement sustainable and not reliant on an external provider to support the client.

There are different interpretations of supported employment and each type of supported employment gives different options and opportunities for the individuals involved. Mobile crews tender for jobs in a community and might consist of 4–8 workers and one supervisor. This set-up is suited to grounds maintenance and house cleaning. The whole work team travel together from job to job and the service provider employs them.

Enclaves are eight or so workers employed in a community-based host business, sometimes employed by the service provider but more often employed by the business itself. These people remain in the same workplace and receive job coaching for part of the day only with the job coach in this service model being an employee of the service provider.

A one-to-one approach is where intensive support is given from a job coach throughout the whole day. The job coach ensures the quality of the work that is being produced by the employee (French Gilson 1998).

In the UK, supported employment seems to be available for some individuals who may be experiencing more complex obstacles to return to work; those who may have a health condition which is longer term and chronic; or for those who may have lifelong disabilities. Providers can be from the voluntary sector, charitable sector, health service, local authority or independent sector.

Evidence-based interventions

'We have sufficient knowledge and evidence to reduce sickness absence and the number of people who go on to long-term incapacity, and to improve job retention, return to work, and reintegration.' (Waddell et al. 2004)

Is there then a paucity of research that proves or disproves the beneficial effects of vocational rehabilitation?

Much of the research describing vocational rehabilitation does exactly this – it describes services rather than providing evidence in the traditional medical sense to prove that it works effectively. The DWP (2004a) said:

'*Currently the evidence is inconclusive about the relative effectiveness and added value of VR (vocational rehabilitation).*'

One reason for this could be the broad definition of vocational rehabilitation and the fact that it relates to many services and not just one intervention. There is an abundance of anecdotal data around, as well as individual case studies, and these are useful from an individual clinical intervention perspective and for service design in a particular area. But what is often required is data that can then be generalised and which shows value for money, especially for commissioners of services. Waddell et al. (2004) in their document *Concepts of Rehabilitation for the Management of Common Health Problems: Evidence Base* show that:

- Since 1943 there have been more than 21 reports relating to UK rehabilitation policy and services.
- Since 1995 there have been more than 26 reviews and guidance on occupational management.
- In recent years there have been:
  - 35 reports and research papers with the main findings from reviews of mental health conditions.
  - 17 research papers with the main findings from reviews of low back pain.
  - 25 research papers with reviews of musculoskeletal conditions (including 'pain').
  - 29 research papers with reviews of cardiorespiratory conditions.

That makes 153 useful pieces of material looking at common health problems and vocational rehabilitation. To date, as the pace of vocational rehabilitation has gained speed and importance in the UK, this number of published papers related to vocational rehabilitation and common health problems is likely to be much higher and this is fantastic news! More and more agencies are recognising the importance of managing common health problems in reducing sickness absence, in job retention and in return to work and as such more useful information is being published.

What evidence do we need about vocational rehabilitation interventions? Figure 4.2 suggests some of the required areas for evidence.

It is far beyond the scope of this book to identify all the evidence and represent it here in a readable format. My advice is for you to:

- Stay up-to-date with who is producing the evidence
- Evaluate the evidence
- Determine how useful it is for your service
- Ensure that everyone in your service knows about the evidence, including, most importantly your service users

You could join relevant groups and associations so that you have a means by which to filter relevant information by reading journals, a wide range of books and reports, attending conferences, web forums, podcasts, email updates and other

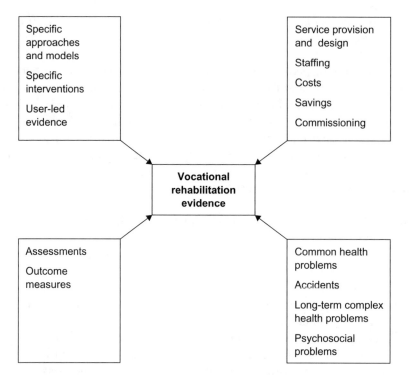

Figure 4.2 Evidence requirements in terms of vocational rehabilitation.

media. Within organisations there are often sub-groups or special interest groups that may be even more relevant to you. Some of the relevant organisations are:

- The College of Occupational Therapists
- The Vocational Rehabilitation Association
- The British Association of Rehabilitation Medicine
- Chartered Society of Physiotherapists
- The Psychological Association
- The British Association of Supported Employment
- The Ergonomics Society
- The various health charities such as
  - Rehab UK
  - Royal National Institute for the Blind
  - Royal National Institute for the Deaf
  - MIND
  - Multiple Sclerosis Society
  - Scope
- The various employment support charities such as:
  - Shaw Trust
  - Remploy

- The Prince's Trust
- Leonard Cheshire
- The various disability organisations:
  - Disability Alliance
  - RADAR
  - The British Council of Disabled People
- Service user groups locally and nationally
- Royal College of Physicians
- Society of Occupational Medicine
- Faculty of Occupational Medicine
- National Institute for Mental Health in England
- Case Management Society UK
- Chartered Institute of Personnel and Development
- Trades Union Congress
- Confederation of British Industry
- Employers' Forum on Disability
- Work and Health Network

This is just a short list of the organisations that you may want to look up to see what they are providing in the way of evidence related to vocational rehabilitation. (Apologies to those organisations I have not mentioned – I have not intentionally left anyone out.) It is also paramount, in my view, to maintain awareness of current government programmes, initiatives, research and policies and the three major departments are the Department of Health, the Department of Work and Pensions and the Health and Safety Executive as well as other units such as the Social Exclusion Unit.

Some of the evidence:

- For vocational rehabilitation with common health problems: Waddell & Burton 2000; Mindout 2002, 2003; van Tulder & Koes 2002; Waddell & Watson 2004
- For vocational rehabilitation with long-term complex problems: Frank et al. 1996, 1998; de Buck et al. 2002; Menz et al. 2003
- For vocational rehabilitation with psychosocial problems: Olsheski et al. 2002
- For vocational rehabilitation for specific approaches: Stuckey 1997; Bond et al. 1998; Baronet & Gerber 1998; Ghates 2000; Haldorson et al. 2002; Thomas et al. 2002; Crowther et al. 2004. These approaches include:
  - Cognitive behavioural approach
  - Individual placement and support (IPS) model of supported employment
  - Case management model
  - Employee assistance programmes
  - Multidisciplinary interventions
  - Industrial-based interventions
- For vocational rehabilitation about specific interventions: Krause et al. 1998; Cox et al. 2000; de Gaudemaris 2000; Feuerstein et al. 2000; Isernhagen 2000;

Brooker et al. 2001; Karsh et al. 2001; Mital & Mital 2002; Pransky et al. 2002; Schonstein et al. 2002; Devereaux 2003; Monninkhof et al. 2003; Nordqvist et al. 2003; Shaw et al. 2003; Thomson et al. 2003; van der Klink & van Dijk 2003. These approaches include:
- Cognitive behavioural psychotherapy
- Self-management education programmes
- Stress management techniques
- Work hardening
- Ergonomics
- Modified work
- Cardiac rehabilitation
- Workplace interventions
- Job simulation
● For service user-led research: Inman et al. 2005/06

The Service User Research Group of England (SURGE) is one of a number of organisations that support service user led research and is the service user arm of the UK Mental Health Research Network (MHRN). SURGE is a national network set up to support mental health service users and people from universities and NHS trusts, as they work together on mental health research.

Timing vocational rehabilitation

Rehabilitation should not be a second stage once treatment has gone as far as medically possible (Waddell et al. 2004) and vocational rehabilitation should not be the tertiary stage to a person's re-integration into society and work:

'It should be integral to good clinical and occupational management.'

Evidence shows that rehabilitation is best started between one and six months off work, although Waddell et al. (2004) say that the exact times are unclear from current evidence. It is understood that if interventions occur earlier than one month, most people will recover naturally and return to work uneventfully. If interventions occur later than six months then the obstacles to return to work become more complex and harder to overcome: rehabilitation is more difficult and costly, and has a lower success rate.

A possible process for vocational rehabilitation

Once you have assessed your client, and their workplace and their functional capacity in whatever ways are appropriate for your service, your interventions may follow the pattern in Table 4.2. The vocational rehabilitation programme and interventions may be offered by your service or you may have to refer your client to another service or contract in specialists. That will depend on your service arrangements. The programmes and interventions that your client will attend may be on

Table 4.2 Potential interventions, service providers and outcomes in a vocational rehabilitation programme.

Action	Potential intervention	Potential service provider	Potential outcome
Establishing the fit of the workplace and job to the individual	Job matching to see how well the job and the individual come together	A service with a suitably experienced practitioner who understands human function (physical and psychological) and understands ergonomics and environments	Specific recommendations for alterations to the job, workplace and recommendations for the individual concerning skills, physical and psychological functioning and self-management
	Welfare rights advice	Case manager	
		Citizens Advice Bureaux	Advice on financial implications of sickness benefits and/or working and/or retirement
		Jobcentre Plus	
		Union reps	
The individual would benefit from some changes	Work conditioning	NHS/PCT (rehab teams)	Increased capacity to undertake physical activity and work tasks
	Work hardening	Some training organisations in the independent sector	
	Self-management techniques (could include family)	Condition management programmes at JCP	Improved self-management of long-term conditions, symptoms, etc.
	Job simulation	Workplace health (OHS, EAP)	Improved confidence and self-efficacy
		Insurance-provided rehab programme	
Some education would be beneficial	Skills in literacy, numeracy, etc. (specialist assistance for dyslexia)	Training organisations	Increased skill base in order to offer a wider range of potential work
	Personal skills in communication, social skills, etc.	NHS/PCT (Rehab teams)	
		Local authority	Improved confidence and self-efficacy
	Practical work skills training	Independent specialist provider	
		Unions	

Table 4.2 *continued.*

Action	Potential intervention	Potential service provider	Potential outcome
The workplace would benefit from some changes	Modification to tools and equipment	Access to Work at JCP	The workplace environment and the people within the workplace are able to confidently include your client
	Modification to workplace environment	NHS/PCT (rehab teams)	
		Workplace health (OHS, EAP, Health and Safety)	
	Education to the workforce (selected people)	Insurance-provided rehab programme	Develop a workplace adjustment plan including reasonable adjustments
		Occupational psychology	
	Cultural shift in the management	Ergonomics service	
		Independent specialist provider	
The client's home would benefit from some changes	Modification to home equipment	NHS/PCT (rehab teams)	The client's home and the important people that he or she interacts with regularly are able to confidently facilitate your client in his or her return to work
	Modification to home environment	Insurance-provided rehab programme	
	Education to the community (selected people)	Local authority	
		Independent specialist provider	
The job task would benefit from some changes	Reorganisation of tasks within a job	NHS/PCT (rehab teams)	The job is adapted to suit the individual for an agreed amount of time (could be permanent)
	Reorganisation of overall hours	Workplace health (OHS, EAP)	
	Reorganisation of start and finish times	Insurance-provided rehab programme	Develop a graded return to work plan together with a monitoring programme
		Psychology	
	Reorganisation of transport to and from work	Ergonomics service	
		Independent specialist provider	
	Alternative duties or new duties	Access to Work at JCP (transport)	

Career mapping and job searching would be beneficial	Career counselling	Independent specialist provider	A clear idea of the type of suitable career in a local area and opportunities for positive experiences of interviews
	Job search skills	Connexions	
	Job interviewing skills (including preparation and performance)	Disability Employment Advisor at JCP	Advice on financial implications of sickness benefits and/or working
	Self-reflection skills	Independent career services (computerised or face-to-face)	
	Welfare rights advice	Job brokers	
		Pathways to Work scheme at JCP	
		Citizens Advice Bureaux, JCP Union reps	
A job placement would be beneficial	Supported placement in paid work	Job Brokers	A successful placement in work of some type, which is appropriate for the client with just the right amount of support
	Supported placement in unpaid work	Pathways to work scheme at JCP	
	Supported meaningful occupation	Disability Employment Advisor at JCP	Develop a graded return to work plan together with a monitoring programme
	Unsupported work in paid or unpaid employment	NHS/PCT (Rehab teams)	
		Independent specialist supported employment provider	Gradual removal of support and follow up plans
		Insurance provided rehab programme	
		LA	
		Community Volunteer Services	
		Unions	

NHS National Health Service (pertaining to secondary care)
PCT Primary Care Trust (pertaining to community care)
OHS Occupational Health Service
EAP Employee Assistance Programme (pertaining to those offered by a workplace)
JCP Job Centre Plus
LA Local Authority (pertaining to support services to young people and adults)

a one-to-one basis e.g. cognitive behavioural psychotherapy or career advice, or in a group e.g. work skills training or self-management techniques.

In the present climate in the UK, the service providers may be qualified rehabilitation professionals, unqualified but experienced practitioners in vocational rehabilitation or completely inexperienced qualified or unqualified practitioners. It would be wise to set up some type of quality measure that you need your service provider to meet, because your client's life does not need to have any more negative influences than they might already have. It would be wise to expect to view all the practitioners' CVs before they see your client, and to check that they are registered with the appropriate regulatory bodies, e.g. Health Professions Council before they start working. As a client you can ask to see and be told about the qualifications and experience that your practitioner has to work with you and if you have reasonable doubt as to their capability, then tell someone.

A case manager who keeps a perspective of the big picture while the client immerses himself or herself in particular interventions may oversee the vocational rehabilitation programme. The pathway to work is not straightforward – it is not always easy to obtain all the right interventions for your client at the right time, yet. But it is important, I believe, to have an idea of the range of services that are available to your client and the potential outcomes that may be on offer to your client. The challenge is not whether your service can attract the right kinds of clients, but whether you can attract the right kinds of services and interventions for your client.

Health and social interventions

The health and social care sector in the UK is quite enormous and spans the NHS, local authorities, voluntary, independent and charitable providers. With regard to vocational rehabilitation, the providers within the sector are still numerous. This section explores some of those providers, and discusses the kinds of professionals and practitioners who are involved and their potential roles, so that you can understand the service or organisation a little more. It will also describe the types of vocational rehabilitation interventions that might be offered, with some resource information to help further research.

National Health Service (NHS)

In England there are 28 strategic health authorities and numerous NHS trusts and mental health trusts. The health services in the devolved countries of Scotland, Wales and Northern Ireland are configured differently from those in England. In Scotland there are 15 health boards covering the country. In Wales there are 22 local health boards that have the same geographical boundaries as the local authorities and Wales has 15 NHS trusts. In Northern Ireland, health and personal social services are provided as an integrated service under four health and social services boards. More information on this is available at:

Northern Ireland   www.n-i.nhs.uk
Scotland   www.scotland.gov.uk
Wales   www.wales.nhs.uk/
England   www.nhs.uk

One part of the NHS that is relevant is known as primary care and this is where the GP works. The other relevant area is secondary care and is usually based in hospitals where patients are acutely ill. There is nationwide coverage of these establishments and patients are seen in various departments, dependent on diagnosis. Vocational rehabilitation as such is not widespread within the NHS, and if it is available it would normally be provided by NHS rehabilitation health professionals as part of the normal hospital rehabilitation services. Some hospitals will have dedicated rehabilitation units with consultants in rehabilitation medicine, but this in itself is no guarantee that vocational rehabilitation will be provided. Some NHS hospitals do provide vocational rehabilitation – Derby Royal Infirmary in Derbyshire and Wexham Park Hospital in Berkshire are two of these.

There may be some elements of vocational rehabilitation, especially with regards to job retention, that occur in the acute stages of a patient's stay in hospital. These may be carried out by a variety of health professions, not just rehabilitation staff.

A few NHS occupational health departments provide a multidisciplinary vocational rehabilitation service but these will be addressed later under workplace interventions.

In the NHS, staffing will vary substantially between hospitals and services. Not every hospital will provide a rehabilitation unit with a rehabilitation physician. Many hospitals will provide therapists for certain wards such as the surgical wards and these therapists will inevitably provide some rehabilitation as this is what they were trained to do (in the UK). Nursing staff may be able to provide support in the functional rehabilitation process while also attending to their other nursing roles. The rehabilitation focused on return to work will likely be superseded by rehabilitation helping an individual return home. Many hospitals provide post-discharge rehabilitation in the form of outpatient services and this – as well as the outreach services – will provide the greatest opportunity for rehabilitation staff and specialist nurses to engage in vocational rehabilitation.

There is no uniformity (in my own experience) in rehabilitation services and this makes it difficult to write about and guide you to understand which professionals and services you and your client might expect to find. That said, NHS facilities in secondary care might have or buy in:

- Occupational therapy services
- Physiotherapy services
- Speech and language services
- Nursing
- Psychology services

Specific rehabilitation units tend to be designed for certain diagnoses or criteria and as such specialist units may have additional staff:

- Prosthetics and orthotics
- Medical physics
- Wheelchair specialists
- Mobility and driving specialists
- Counselling and psychotherapy
- Specialist nurses in conditions such as multiple sclerosis, Parkinson's disease or epilepsy
- Employment specialists

Currently the focus of the NHS, on the whole, is about rehabilitation to facilitate safe discharge from hospital and in these terms, return to work may not be an immediate priority. However, the seeds can be sown and work can be discussed easily, signposting can occur to assist the patient post-discharge and communication with employers, Jobcentre Plus, insurance companies, etc. can be carried out in the same way that liaison might take place with an equipment supplier. In the specialist rehabilitation services, the outreach services and the outpatient services, the scope is further enhanced because the individual is closer to the community, going home regularly (or at home/work) and getting back into a normal routine.

Really there is a wealth of expertise already within the acute hospitals that could advise and facilitate patients to keep their jobs and return to them.

Primary care trusts (PCT)

These are the community services provided through GP surgeries and other community-based services that are commissioned by a PCT. Vocational rehabilitation may be provided as part of a rehabilitation service such as a multidisciplinary brain injury service. Although there are PCTs that cover the UK, the vocational rehabilitation services they provide, as with secondary care, is not uniformly available. It would be fair to say that some geographical areas will have better provision than others and, generally speaking, the mental health services will have the more established vocational rehabilitation services and links with local providers of vocational rehabilitation.

In the PCTs there is a focus on community care and rehabilitation with some small hospitals also providing care. The community arena is much closer to the workplace than the acute hospital and certainly GPs will be addressing work and health issues with their patients daily. The GP has a pivotal role in return to work. Under the NHS Terms of Service they are to:

'Provide advice, to their patients about whether, as a result of a medical disease or disablement, the patient should refrain from their usual type of work.'
(Chambers et al. 2001)

This will include a range of duties including signing people 'off sick' and signing them 'back to work' again. The 'sick note' that the GP writes is an official document that is recognised as medical evidence that the patient cannot do their normal occupation. An employer or the Department for Work and Pensions can accept the sick note as such evidence.

The GP might be the only person someone sees when they are off sick and GPs have the opportunity to signpost patients to appropriate vocational rehabilitation services locally. The GP is also in a prime situation to start giving the patient positive messages about work and health (if indeed work would not compromise a person's health, which in some situations may be the case).

Chambers et al. (2001) suggest that the practice nurse also has a role in addressing chronic illness and disability in relation to fitness to work.

The health visitor has a role in supporting clients' decisions regarding returning to work, e.g. mothers returning to work following maternity leave who may have postnatal conditions, or disabled mothers wanting to return to work after childbirth.

Many GP surgeries have a practice physiotherapist. In a similar way to the GP, the physio has a captive audience of people who may be struggling at work or off sick with musculoskeletal problems and pain. They are in an optimum position to give well-placed advice about working and returning to work as well as sending those positive messages about health and work. However, like most of the practitioners in the GP surgery, the appointment slots are quite short and there is often a full list of people to be seen at every session. This can cause a tension between what can feasibly be accomplished in a session and what the practitioner might want to achieve regarding return to work help.

There are community rehabilitation teams of different types in some PCTs and these can comprise a similar group of practitioners as commonly seen in the hospitals. Their remit can often be to provide post-hospital rehabilitation for a limited period of time and based around personal safety and independence, but also addressing community integration. There may be more scope already for these teams to be involved in vocational rehabilitation and arguably opportunities too. The team may be mobile and able to see people at home, so why not at work? Independence for adults in most instances would include work of some sort and the older adult that many community teams see would not necessarily be out of work just because they have passed their so-called retirement age.

The surgery may have an employment specialist available, who can see people to give them advice about work and health. There are a number of GP surgeries providing this service now and Sheffield is one city that has being doing so successfully for a number of years. Their model is based on the local PCTs providing grants for services from an organisation called Sheffield Occupational Health and Advisory Service (SOHAS), which is a charity.

NHS expert patient programmes

The expert patient programme (EPP) is organised under the NHS and consists of specially trained expert patients and service users who conduct a range of health promotion and education. The Expert Patients website (www.expertpatients. nhs.uk) says:

> 'Patient self-management or "Expert Patient" programmes are not simply about educating patients about their condition or giving them relevant information – they are based on developing patients' confidence and motivation to use their own skills, information and professional services to take effective control over life with a chronic condition.'

The newest initiative is the development of the EPP community interest company (CIC) established to market and deliver the EPP to better meet the needs of people in marginalised and vulnerable groups. While EPPs do not specifically address issues around working with long-term health conditions, they do address taking control of one's life and choosing priorities in which to engage – and work may be one of these priorities.

Local authorities

By local authorities I mean county councils and district councils. There is UK-wide coverage of two-tier county councils and local government departments within them. County councils are responsible for countywide issues including social services and education. Information regarding local authorities is available through the websites of county and district councils as well as Directgov (www.direct.gov.uk). District councils are responsible for issues at a more local level, including housing.

England	36 counties
Northern Ireland	6 counties
Scotland	32 council areas
Wales	9 counties

Major urban areas have a one-tier system called borough councils or metropolitan district councils and other areas have opted for unitary authorities that are also single-tier systems.

Scotland, Wales and Northern Ireland have devolved governments and as such have their authorities arranged in slightly different ways. Scottish and Welsh councils continue to provide social services, whereas Northern Ireland's social services are integrated with health services.

Support workers, healthcare professionals and social interventions professionals carry out vocational rehabilitation with clients who generally are not acutely ill and who have long-term conditions. Teams tend to be arranged around very broad age bands, and interventions will normally still occur in diagnosis-based services such as learning disabilities or sensory impairments. Teachers and tutors in this sector play a large part in preparing young people for work through the wide-ranging curricula they offer at secondary education level.

The majority of the vocational rehabilitation practitioners in the local authority would sit under social services. Occupational therapists work in local authorities and they traditionally have a large part of their time taken up with assessing for adaptive equipment and adaptations to properties occupied by disabled people. But many occupational therapists will provide advice to people who are working or want to return to work and this is a legitimate part of their role.

Community support workers will have a role in facilitating their clients in their everyday tasks, and work may be one of the activities.

Social workers can have a wide range of roles with their clients, depending on their clients' needs. They may take a role in managing a client's care and ensuring that all the relevant services are involved. This care management role may involve referrals to services to support people into work and in preparing people for work.

'Social work is a human rights discipline – social workers work with people to achieve social welfare, social justice and social inclusion – where that is sought by the individual.' (British Association of Social Workers, www.basw.co.uk)

Care trusts

These are not primary care trusts but are a type of NHS body introduced in 2002 to provide better-integrated health and social interventions. By combining both NHS responsibilities and local authority health responsibilities under a single management, care trusts can increase continuity of care and simplify administration. Care trusts are set up when the NHS and local authorities agree to work closely together, usually where it is felt that a closer relationship between health and social interventions is needed or would benefit local care services (Department of Health, NHS England 2006). There are currently nine care trusts in England. Sheffield Care Trust is one such NHS care trust that has a thriving vocational rehabilitation service in the mental health division, together with a consultant occupational therapist responsible for vocational rehabilitation.

Health charities

According to the Charity Commission a charity is an organisation

'set up for exclusively charitable purposes which carries out activities to achieve these purposes. A charity must be set up to help the public and not particular individuals.'

Charitable purposes can be broken down into these four main categories:

- Relief of financial hardship, old age, sickness or disability
- Advancement of education
- Advancement of religion
- Other charitable purposes which help and benefit the community

On the Charity Commission website (www.charity-commission.gov.uk) there are more than 167 500 charities in England and Wales (as of end June 2006). Over 500 charitable organisations were listed when I searched for 'health' and when I searched for 'disability' there were 200 entries, and 35 results emerged from searching for 'vocational rehabilitation'. The equivalent organisation in Scotland is the Office of the Scottish Charity Regulator (OSCR) and in Northern Ireland it is the Department for Social Development (DSD). Not all the charities on the website provide a service in the UK, but it is astounding just how many relevant charities there are and how many may provide health and social support for people looking at training, education and working.

Many charities have been developed to help people with particular impairments, conditions and diagnoses such as:

- Multiple Sclerosis Society
- RNIB (Royal National Institute of the Blind)
- MIND
- Rehab UK
- Royal MENCAP Society
- Spinal Injuries Association

There are those charities that deal with the broader issues of disability such as:

- Leonard Cheshire Foundation
- Dial UK
- Motability
- Disability Information Service

And there are those that deal with working, such as:

- Association of Disabled Professionals
- Employment Opportunities for People with Disabilities
- Shaw Trust

Volunteer organisations

Volunteering England defines volunteering as

> 'any activity that involves spending time, unpaid, doing something that aims to benefit the environment or someone (individuals or groups) other than, or in addition to, close relatives. Central to this definition is the fact that volunteering must be a choice freely made by each individual.' (www.volunteering.org.uk)

Voluntary organisations can be found all over the UK and many will be charities as well:

- The National Council for Voluntary Organisations (www.ncvo-vol.org.uk): Umbrella body for the voluntary sector in England
- The Scottish Council for Voluntary Organisations (www.scvo.org.uk): National body representing the voluntary sector
- Wales Council for Voluntary Action (www.wcva.org.uk): Represents, supports and campaigns for volunteers, voluntary organisations and communities in Wales
- The Volunteer Development Agency in Northern Ireland (www.volunteering-ni.org): Support, training and information on volunteering, volunteer management, child protection and voluntary management committees

Voluntary organisations are important in supporting return to work programmes and in supporting individuals. Well established programmes such as those provided by the Forestry Commission, RNIB or the National Trust provide working opportunities that an individual might not otherwise be able to get in paid employment. In England the Do It website (www.do-it.org.uk) provides the opportunities to search for vacancies in volunteering, and Scotland has the Volunteer Scotland website (www.volunteerscotland.org.uk). Wales has Volunteering Wales (www.volunteering-wales.net) showing vacancies for volunteers and Northern Ireland has the Volunteer Development Agency (www.volunteering-ni.org) which signposts people to each of the regions to enquire about vacancies. Some of these opportunities may be about supporting people into work as a role for a volunteer or in providing work for people.

Another useful organisation has part of its website identified for locating projects that are related to vocational rehabilitation and return to work but which may be charitable, voluntary, of statutory provision or independent. On The Side is a charity which mainly supports the efforts of small user-led mental health groups (www.ontheside.org). One of the sections on its website is a list of employment projects around the UK (www.ontheside.org/direct). The website describes the set-up of the project:

'In 2001 the University of York's Social Policy Research Unit carried out a survey for the Department of Work and Pensions which analysed data for 2520 disability-focused employment projects. 937 of these cater for people with mental health problems (or another disability). 1538 of them cater for mental health problems or with learning difficulties. The remaining 982 projects focus on other disabilities.'

I use this resource often to locate suitable opportunities for my own clients. On The Side attempts to update the information when it has the resources to do so.

Smaller groups and projects like the Heeley City Farm project in Sheffield, South Yorkshire provide work experience, supported employment and open employment opportunities.

Within the charity and voluntary sector there is a wide profile of practitioners, from those who have multiple higher education qualifications to those who have no qualifications per se and have a wealth of experience – and then those in between.

You can expect to see many health professionals, social interventions practitioners, support workers, welfare advisors, case managers and careers advisors. This wide variety of experience of people with such a range of qualifications helps to make this sector flexible to people's needs, often providing very pertinent services. However, as with any practitioner you should check whether the person who is dealing with your client or you as the consumer has the correct 'qualifications' to carry out vocational rehabilitation and return to work support.

- Does the service provide you with a résumé of the skills and experience of the practitioner they are suggesting your client works with?
- What assurances do they provide regarding the quality of the work that is carried out in their project or service?

Department for Work and Pensions (DWP) and Department of Health (DH)

The DWP document *Pathways to Work: Qualitative Research on the Condition Management Programmes* (Barnes & Hudson 2006) describes the condition management programmes (CMP) initiated as a result of the Pathways to Work Green Paper in 2002. These programmes are part of wider changes that were made to claimants of Incapacity Benefit (IB) in particular pilot areas in the UK. The pilots commenced in 2003 over three Jobcentre Plus districts and then this was extended by four more districts in 2004. As part of the welfare reforms it is hoped to roll out this programme to all Jobcentre districts. The first seven areas were:

- Renfrewshire, Inverclyde, Argyll and Bute
- Essex
- Derbyshire
- East Lancashire
- Somerset
- Bridgend and Rhondda Cynon Taf
- Gateshead and South Tyneside

CMPs are work-focused and part of the *Choices Package* of interventions in the Pathways to Work Scheme, and offer support to people returning to work. Jobcentre Plus and local NHS providers in a given area provide CMPs jointly. CMPs are a voluntary element to Pathways to Work and 'customers' (people claiming IB) are referred to the programme via their IB Personal Advisor (IBPA). The programmes provide brief interventions about managing one's health and lifestyle to facilitate return to work and are carried out in groups and in one-to-one sessions.

CMPs are an important step in the realisation that health and work are not two separate entities managed by separate silos of services. They show that it is possible for health providers to sit along side Jobcentre Plus staff to facilitate people back into work in an individualised programme that meets a customer's needs.

The teams include occupational therapists, physiotherapists, nurses, cognitive behavioural therapists, occupational psychologists, health psychologists, occupational health nurses and generic practitioners.

Independent providers

The term independent provider is used in this book to refer to those organisations or individuals who provide vocational rehabilitation and are not charities, statutory services or the voluntary sector. That leaves specific companies, partnerships and sole traders that are set up to make independent earnings from providing services. Within the sector of health and social interventions these independent providers (of which I am currently one) will be dominated by health professionals and can be seen in Table 4.3.

Insurance companies

Insurance companies in the UK are a growing provider/purchaser of health and social interventions rehabilitation with an ultimate aim of returning a person to paid employment. The Association of British Insurers says:

> 'The insurance industry spends £2 bn a year on healthcare – money that would otherwise have to come from the NHS.' (ABI 2005)

Rehabilitation can be provided for some policyholders in the UK when they take out insurance policies for (for example):

- Employers' liability
- Personal accident
- Income protection and critical illness
- Health
- Employee assistance programmes

Some insurance companies provide in-house services, such as Unum Provident, which employs rehabilitation staff. Others, such as NFU Mutual, buy in or have independent associates that provide rehabilitation services. If you or your client want to research whether they could be engaged in rehabilitation through their insurance provider, then talk to the claims handler for their case, or the solicitor if there is one involved.

The range of practitioners and health and social care professionals in the independent sector mirrors to a great extent what is available in the public services. However, rather than being bounded by postcodes these services are often available countrywide. The idea is not necessarily to duplicate existing services but often to plug a gap and to provide something that was not there to start with or available in a timely fashion.

Table 4.3 Independent providers of vocational rehabilitation.

Provider type	How to find them	Website
Physiotherapy companies and individual chartered physiotherapists	Physio First is the organisation of Chartered Physiotherapists in Private Practice, which has approximately 4000 members	www.physiofirst.org.uk
	Association of Chartered Physiotherapists in Occupational Health and Ergonomics is a specialist interest group recognised by the Chartered Society of Physiotherapy founded in 1947	www.acpohe.org.uk
Occupational therapy companies and individual occupational therapists	College of Occupational Therapists Specialist Section: Independent Practice (OTIP) is the specialist section of occupational therapists in independent practice. There is also a free phone telephone number	www.otip.co.uk Helpline 0800 389 4873
	College of Occupational Therapists specialist interest group for work	www.cot.org.uk
Psychology-based companies and individual psychologists of different types	British Psychological Society website has a comprehensive search to find psychologists	www.bps.org.uk
Private or independent hospitals	Dr Foster website provides a search for all the NHS and private hospitals in the UK	www.drfoster.co.uk
Cognitive behavioural therapy companies and individuals who are qualified to practice in CBT	The British Association of Behavioural and Cognitive Psychotherapies website has a comprehensive search to find accredited therapists	www.babcp.com
Rehabilitation companies	The most comprehensive list of providers that people can search to find the right organisation for their client or themselves is Rehabwindow. This is a web based information portal and directory listing rehabilitation services and products.	www.rehabwindow.net
	European Platform for Rehabilitation website lists organisations that have met the requirements of the EQRM (European Quality in Rehabilitation Mark)	www.epr.be
Case management companies and individual case managers, who will normally come from a health or social care profession	Case Management Society of the UK is the society for case managers practising in all fields, including vocational rehabilitation. They can provide a service to find a case manager	www.cmsuk.org
	The British Association of Brain Injury Case Managers is the professional association for case management in the field of acquired brain injury. They provide a list of UK members and contact details	www.babicm.org

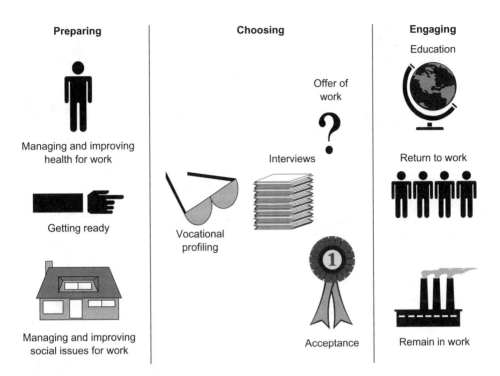

Preparing

Managing and improving
health for work

Getting ready

Managing and improving
social issues for work

Choosing

Offer of
work

Interviews

Vocational
profiling

Acceptance

Engaging

Education

Return to work

Remain in work

Figure 4.3 A mind map to help structure vocational rehabilitation interventions.
Images from Microsoft Clip Art.

Types of interventions in health and social interventions

I have seen many different flow charts and diagrams that attempt to demonstrate the processes and access points for a pathway to work that requires vocational rehabilitation. I have not yet found one comprehensive enough to show all the possible scenarios in which clients might find themselves and yet simple enough to understand. However, the interventions that are possible in vocational rehabilitation are likely to continue to be a complicated topic that is difficult to dissect and explain. This is partly because there are so many organisations providing vocational rehabilitation in an unregulated and unmapped field and partly because vocational rehabilitation is a complex set of interventions, different for each individual.

To provide some structure to the process of describing the interventions, I have provided a mind map in Figure 4.3 of how I see vocational rehabilitation in the UK, which is based on my experiences with clients. This may not be wholly appropriate for you and your client, but the purpose here is just to provide a structure by which to describe the interventions rather than a particular evidence-based pathway.

Interventions can be thought of as being broadly part of preparing for entering work, part of choosing work and part of engaging in work. In preparing for

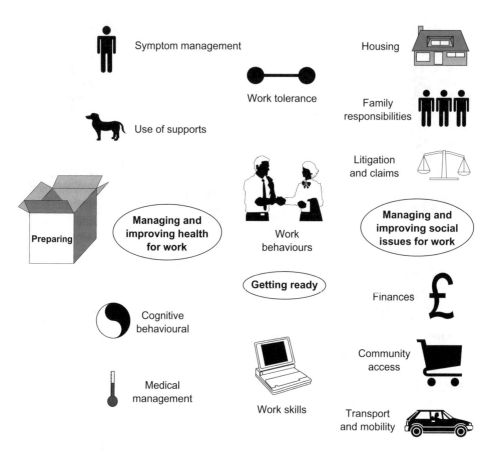

Figure 4.4 Preparing for work: health and social interventions.
Images from Microsoft Clip Art.

work, the interventions could be subdivided into managing and improving health for work, into getting ready for work and into managing and improving social issues for work.

In choosing work the interventions could be subdivided into vocational profiling, into interviews, into obtaining an offer of work and into acceptance of a work offer.

In engaging in work the interventions can be subdivided into engaging with education, into engaging in returning to work or entering work and into remaining in work.

Figure 4.4 now expands the first part of the mind map by suggesting in more detail the interventions that one might expect to find in preparing for work, which tend to fall under health and social care interventions. There are no definite boundaries in vocational rehabilitation in the UK and in many ways this makes it less rigid than it might be otherwise.

The sector of health and social interventions has a long history of preparing and supporting people to live in the community and with regards to considering a working life this provision remains important. Working – whether it is voluntary or paid – is likely to be much more difficult if your client is having difficulty managing their health condition or if their local community is causing them to be disabled; or if your client has not yet attained the stamina to go to work. In my experience of working in health and social interventions, this sector is already part way to preparing their clients/patients/customers for some future work but is lacking some focus on this goal in some areas. Certainly for many people, getting out of hospital is only the first stage of a recovery process and not the ultimate goal, which for a lot of people would be about attaining some quality of life that might be gained through work of some sort (not necessarily paid or work in a traditional sense). The kinds of intervention that might be considered in this preparation phase can be described under the following headings:

- Managing and improving health for work
  - Medical management
  - Symptom management
  - Cognitive and behavioural management
  - Use of supports
- Getting ready for work
  - Work tolerance
  - Work behaviours
  - Work skills
- Managing and improving social issues for work
  - Housing
  - Family responsibilities
  - Litigation and claims
  - Finances
  - Community access
  - Transport and mobility

Managing and improving health for work

Medical management

By medical management I mean the intervention and monitoring that the doctor, nurse or other health professional provides in ameliorating health conditions. Without wanting to state the obvious, the immediate health needs that people face should be addressed as a primary concern to ease suffering and possible further loss of function or life. So the medical interventions are sometimes necessary. An orthopaedic surgeon will be able to perform surgery to pin and plate someone's broken leg, without which the individual might be left with nerve damage, long-term pain and a shortened limb. While these interventions do not directly relate to the workplace (often), they serve an important role in helping people manage their health condition. However, how healthcare is managed and appointments arranged, for instance, can impact directly on someone getting back to work. Often clients worry about going back to work and then disrupt routines with colleagues at work by coming away for appointments to see health professionals for ongoing treatment or consultations. Out-of-hours services, including those at weekends, can make a dramatic difference to a person's feeling of control over their health and work situation.

Managing medication is also an important element of having control over a health condition or symptoms. But mismanagement of medication can have devastating effects for individuals. Understanding the medication that someone requires to maintain health is often addressed by nurses and doctors, who are in turn often guided by pharmacists. Some medication can have a dramatic effect on a person's ability to drive or operate machinery safely and alternative drugs may be available to prescribe. It is only if the health professional asks about whether the individual is working or wanting to return to work that these issues can be avoided.

Careful monitoring from specialist nurses and specialist teams can mean that people with long-term conditions such as multiple sclerosis or arthritis can potentially remain in a job that they enjoy and feel satisfied with rather than losing it. It is important for the individual with the health condition to feel in control of their life and their work situation.

Symptom management

This could include education-based programmes that help people become aware of their health condition and take control of their life. Examples of this would be the expert patient programme in the NHS and the condition management programme at Jobcentre Plus. These programmes might be based on particular approaches and theories such as the cognitive behavioural approach. Condition management has been described as

> *'individual intervention to help customers manage their health condition and overcome negative beliefs about work.' (Grove 2005)*

It includes cognitive/educational interventions with elements that are common to all conditions and coping styles and methods.

Specific rehabilitation interventions may be used to help clients overcome particular symptoms and to learn coping strategies. Some examples of these would be anxiety management, stress management, depression management, pain management and joint protection. If you are a clinician you will be able to identify more specific management programmes for the particular symptoms your clients report. These programmes have an educational element to them and they have elements that involve behavioural change and cognitive change. In other words, if you need to be able to work and you have some interfering symptoms, there may be some coping strategies that can be learned that may make living with the symptom easier. This may involve altering some routines and also involve recognising certain behaviours, thoughts and feelings to help create the right environment to learn a new strategy.

The specialist nurses and teams will also have a large part in symptom management and education, especially for people who are newly diagnosed. Many teams will already have a focus on helping their clients to manage their symptoms at work and give advice about such concerns as disclosure of health conditions to employers. They may also take a more active role in communicating with an employer, the human resources department or the occupational health department to liaise between the client and work. An even more active role would be to go into the workplace and to advise on changes that may be appropriate, or to offer awareness training about a health condition. This can have a positive effect in reducing anxieties and problem solving reasonably simple issues, such as appropriate duties, time off for medical appointments and adaptations to a workspace. The teams may also be able to signpost people to other relevant services in the community, such as local job brokers, voluntary work organisations and Access to Work. All these interventions are important in maintaining someone in work and in supporting people to return to work, if that is their choice.

Cognitive and behavioural management

Certain types of issues that may interfere with working may be addressed in a more structured way that requires the client to approach his or her life in a different way to maintain some independence and control. Someone may benefit from more extensive psychotherapy, cognitive behavioural psychotherapy, or psychological intervention such as neuropsychology to comprehensively address the issues that they are faced with. These sorts of intervention need to be provided by a suitably qualified practitioner.

Cognitive rehabilitation may be appropriate for some clients with brain injuries and this can be used to help the client practise those functions of the brain such as memory or visual processing that have been damaged (Japp 2005). This usually occurs at the same time as teaching the client coping strategies and using external prompts for memory, diaries, checklists and learning to use electronic devices such as a mobile phone. These external devices can help an individual learn to become independent and regain some control over his or her life.

Sometimes emotional issues need to be addressed and these may be related to anger over injuries sustained in an accident, not adjusting to lower ability levels and changes in life circumstances. There will be other emotional issues and individual reactions to these differ and as such may respond better to different types of intervention. But with regards to vocational rehabilitation, the outcome of the intervention is to facilitate greater control over one's life to cope with the emotional difficulties and consider working or remain in work. This may include using tools, such as activity diaries, graded exposure and thought diaries. Specific work could include (Macdonald 2004):

- Learning new skills and coping strategies
- Reducing 'excessive' or unhelpful behaviours
- Overcoming avoidance
- Challenging unhelpful ways of thinking and learning new ones
- Reaching a shared understanding
- Engaging the person in the process of change

Behavioural changes may be required in people's routines and habits to maximise functional independence and to get ready for returning to work. A common routine change that I have seen is altered sleep patterns, with clients going to bed in the early hours of the morning and then not waking until midday. While this behaviour is relevant for some types of work it is not relevant for daytime work and this routine often needs restructuring before considering returning to work. There will be many other routines or behaviours that may not facilitate a person returning to work, and these may need to be addressed prior to returning to work and cognitive behavioural techniques is one approach that is used to achieve these changes.

Use of supports

Certain issues cannot be overcome through learning new techniques alone and your client may benefit from using extra supports at home and in their community (supports in the workplace will be addressed later in the chapter). These might be in the form of:

- Environmental adaptations
- Adaptive equipment or assistive technology
- Personal assistants (including animal assistants)

Environmental adaptations in this context would refer to those that help the individual prepare to return to work and would most commonly refer to home and community adaptations. An example might be a ramp to the external doors in a property and a marked disabled parking bay on the road outside the property. This could in turn facilitate the person to get out of the home and get into their vehicle to drive to work. The local authority occupational therapists would assess for this type of adaptation, along with the housing department if the funding sources were to come from the local authority. Likewise, adaptations to other parts of a person's property and garden may help someone become more independent and able to consider getting up for work again and so are important preparations.

Assistive technology can be defined as

'any product or service designed to enable independence for disabled and older people.' (King's Fund Consultation, 14th March 2001 available at the Foundation for Assistive Technology (FAST) www.fastuk.org)

The device may be very high-tech, such as a palm-based computer, or low-tech, such as a plastic tube to build up the circumference of a pen. The actual range of services and equipment is vast and can represent almost all parts of a person's daily activities. The field includes orthotics and prosthetics, communication, computing, equipment manufacturers and retailers and healthcare professionals. There is further education available across the country in different colleges and universities up to Masters level and including informal one-day courses as well from individual manufacturers. FAST includes a database on its website that details all the available courses.

In health and social care the assistive technology that might be arranged will usually come from one of the rehabilitation professionals. The technology may assist a client's In-order-to analysis of their needs for mobility, personal care, communication, literacy needs or childcare. The equipment may be available as part of the statutory provision, or the client may have to pay for it or part of it. It is best to obtain this information from the local community equipment service, which is usually a joint NHS and local authority-run service (Health Act 1999 Section 31 Partnership Agreement for Pooled Fund and Lead Commissioning). The NHS and local authority will provide equipment for use in a person's home and not, so I understand, outside the home.

Personal assistants are sometimes a more suitable help for people than equipment for some activities. Assistants can be available to help with personal care and domestic duties. There are many ways of obtaining help – and help around the home and with personal care is arranged through a care manager within social services for statutory provision. Outside of the statutory provision there are numerous agencies with carers and assistants.

Dogs can also provide assistance. Guide Dogs for the Blind and Hearing Dogs for Deaf People are well-known, but there are other charities that will provide dogs to facilitate independence with their owners who may have a range of independence needs. Further information about these services can be obtained from Support Dogs (www.support-dogs.org.uk) and Canine Partners (www.caninepartners.co.uk).

Getting ready for work

Grading interventions

Grading interventions is important because it reflects the need to make interventions fit individuals rather than a one-size-fits-all approach. In addition grading can be useful for clients to reduce the dependence that individual may feel they have on a service.

Stewart and Wheeler (2005) describe using a graded structure:

'in order to facilitate this growth of awareness and responsibility.'

Many practitioners in health and social interventions would believe that it is right to facilitate independence in their clients – in many cases this would involve a gradual reduction of input in terms of service provision or interventions to a client. Certainly from a business perspective, it would be difficult in the long term to provide a service to an increasing caseload of clients who required ongoing interventions and retain quality in the service.

Stewart and Wheeler (2005) describe how grading is used with group interventions.

'Grading is defined by the role of the facilitators, who gradually withdraw their direction and support until eventually group members can find their needs met through self-help and voluntary groups.'

Table 4.4 Grading a task using self-efficacy theory.

Step 1	To help your client manage the emotional anxiety (arousal) associated with considering the task
Step 2	To verbally encourage and persuade the client that he has the capability of doing the task (not the same as forcing someone to do something against their will)
Step 3	To arrange for your client to see another receptionist doing the same task
Step 4	Arranging for your client to practise the task itself

They are referring to their clients who they see in the community mental health team as they are helping people to develop their occupational identity.

Willard and Spackman (Blesedell Crepeau et al. 2003) define grading as to:

'sequentially increase or decrease the demands of an activity over time to stimulate improvement in the client's function or respond to diminishing functional capacity.'

In psychological interventions, the term 'graded exposure' is used. This means gradually and in a safe manner to lead the client into situations that they find difficult to cope with. Part of the intervention is to show or teach the client how to cope with difficult situations.

This approach uses some concepts from self-efficacy theory to gradually improve someone's beliefs about himself or herself. In self-efficacy, grading comes from designing interventions in such a way as to facilitate the positive experiences gained. For example, if you had a client who wanted to be a receptionist, you might help him to believe that he had the capacity to do the task of answering the telephone and taking a message by following a graded approach. Table 4.4 demonstrates how this might be arranged using self-efficacy theory.

At each stage, according to self-efficacy theory, your client's belief in their ability would increasingly be reinforced and become stronger. So, discussing the task and being verbally persuaded to take a telephone call and a message will not have as much effect on the client as seeing another receptionist or client doing the same task.

Grading can occur in terms of physical activities as well. This is something that we would all be aware of if, for instance, we started to do fell running for the first time. Our muscles and cardiovascular system require time to adjust to increasing physical demands of tasks. In terms of work these physical demands will relate to load, pace and duration and this is often addressed by physiotherapists and occupational therapists in health and social care through general rehabilitation programmes, work conditioning and work hardening.

Work tolerance

Work tolerance is concerned with addressing the individual's ability to endure the requirements of a job in a timely and appropriate manner (Northern Ireland Committee of Occupational Therapists 1992 in Pratt & Jacobs 1997). These programmes have to be conscious of health and safety, primarily because the client is being asked to work harder and harder to make improvements. The client requires frequent monitoring throughout the sessions. Heart rate, blood pressure and other signs may need checking and recording at regular intervals. The client's GP or consultant should have the opportunity to agree with the programme and to set medical parameters if required. The rehabilitation team needs to liaise closely with the doctor. Parameters may include keeping the pulse rate below a certain level or limiting weights to be lifted. These limitations need to be recorded and adhered to and regularly reviewed with the client and the rehabilitation team.

The rehabilitation addressing work tolerance would involve work conditioning. This is similar to a fitness programme and involves non-specific job simulation work tasks. Specific exercises would look at:

- Strengthening
- Flexibility
- Symptom control work on anxiety, pain, depression
- Increasing daily activities
- Increasing activity tolerance generally

In a purist sense, *work conditioning* is intensive goal-oriented rehabilitation to improve physical functioning. It would also involve education and coaching and may cover some symptom management work. It would be constructed so that a client attends the facility for half a day 2–3 times per week for a minimum of three weeks.

Work hardening is job-specific physical and psychological tasks replicating critical aspects of the client's job or elements from the range of tasks that would be expected of the client in a whole day's work. It would usually build up to tolerating a full work shift as per the client's job. In the USA a client can expect to go to a work hardening facility up to 5 days per week for up to 8 hours per day and the programmes would tend to last for between 3 and 12 weeks. Work hardening is concerned with grading activity to improve overall functioning with real or simulated work tasks. It usually requires a team approach and preferably an interdisciplinary team approach.

The main idea with these programmes is to help people become 'work ready'. These programmes can run in conjunction with a phased or graded return to work plan so the person attends work two days per week and the rest of the time he or she is at work hardening. In the USA there is less of an acceptance to 'rest' between work days when on a phased return to work because the attitude is that the person should be working towards attaining their maximum functioning level – not stopping just because they are on a phased return to work.

How does this concept sit with you and your clients?

Why might someone return to work on a phased programme and still rest between days?

In reality many places would not artificially split work conditioning and work hardening rehabilitation options and would provide a seamless transition between the two. I always see the work conditioning part as preparing someone for doing work simulation or real work with some restrictions.

Work simulation relies on a sound job analysis and functional assessment of your client. Work itself is always going to be a better option than work hardening but job simulation can be a safe step towards entering the workplace. Job simulation has good face validity and looks at critical demands of a job. It isn't always necessary to simulate the whole job – there may only be certain parts that are posing a difficulty and it is those parts that may benefit from simulation. The job simulation can be project-based (as in producing items such as those that used to be produced in occupational therapy heavy workshops).

In a similar way to circuit training in a gym, individually designed work circuits provide the job simulation. This would occur after a set of preceding tasks such as:

- Warm-up
- Specific exercise programme (physical, relaxation, concentration, anxiety management)
- Conditioning work (treadmill, bikes, stepper, brisk walking)
- Work hardening (lifting tasks, typing tasks, answering the phone tasks)
- Body mechanics/positioning
- Job simulation

The aim would be to grade the programme by gradually increasing the job simulation circuits and decreasing the exercise elements.

Throughout all of the work tolerance training, techniques can be utilised to teach clients how to control their symptoms for work. One way – activity control of symptoms – is described by Matheson (2002) and remembered by the letters SAMS:

Stop
Assess your activity
Modify what you are doing to improve the situation
Start the activity again

Work behaviours

This would involve adaptation of behaviours associated with working.

These were described in Table 2.8 in relation to assessments and can be divided into work attitudes, work habits and work traits.

Work attitudes are those values that a person may have about work and the strength of a worker role that someone may feel as well as ambitions and motivation to work. These elements may be addressed in group settings to help to make people explicitly aware of how these attitudes can help or hinder a person in their return to work goal. On an individual basis, the client may find it beneficial to explore these issues to become more aware of the behaviours that might stem from the attitudes that they hold.

Work habits are those behaviours that an employer would like to see exhibited in their employee. They are generally thought of as helpful behaviours to the workplace and would include such things as punctuality, safety consciousness, accuracy in work, regular attendance at work and politeness. Programmes that specifically address these positive behaviours for the workplace may offer workplace experience sessions and feedback sessions, videoing the client in a workplace and then describing the positive behaviours and those that may need to be addressed. Peer feedback on behaviour can be a strong influence to behavioural acceptance and change. All of these approaches are looking to improve a client's insight into their behaviour to give them a chance to change. Sometimes the behaviour that needs altering is not the one at work but the one that occurs at home but affects work. Adaptation of routines at home for work, such as getting up at a regular time and going to bed at a reasonable time, can help with attendance and punctuality. Eating breakfast can ensure that the client has sufficient energy to make it until lunchtime. It is not rocket science, just common sense most of the time.

Work traits are the characteristics of a person such as how reliable they are, how much responsibility they show, how much self-confidence they have, how much initiative they demonstrate. The word trait indicates that these elements are fixed and inherent in some way. However, I am not so sure that some of the traits cannot be changed. Through the combination of behaviour modification techniques and other appropriate interventions these elements of a person's behaviour may alter.

Work skills

These can be defined as the psychomotor and social skills related to the demands of employment (Northern Ireland Committee of College of Occupational Therapists 1992). Work skills can be seen in relation to the physical demands of a job, the demands that data place on people, people and things at work and temporal demands. These categories of work skills have been used for many years in the USA to guide job specifications. Table 4.5 lists the skills in relation to data, people and things.

Not mentioned in this list are the softer skills that are also required in workplaces. These would be seen as coming under the category of *work behaviours* and would include such dimensions as social skills and interpersonal communication.

Table 4.5 Skills in relation to data, people and things.

Data	People	Things
Synthesising	Advising/counselling	Setting up
Co-ordinating	Negotiating	Precision working
Analysing	Instructing	Operating–controlling
Compiling	Supervising	Driving–operating
Computing	Diverting	Manipulating–operating
Copying	Persuading	Tending
Comparing	Speaking–signalling	Feeding–operating
	Serving	Handling

Hallam and Leach, in Pratt and Jacobs (1997) explain that the ability to handle social relationships is thought to be more crucial than the possession of task skills in successfully helping people with mental health problems into work. They go on to make the observation that work is a social activity and even in self-employment, it is unlikely these days that there will be no need for some kind of communication and social interaction. Health and social care practitioners in the statutory and non-statutory sectors currently work with people to improve these skills. People with a wide range of health issues will be helped with both physical and mental health concerns.

Improving or gaining new practical work skills related to particular industries is often carried out by the education sector at further education colleges and higher education establishments where some qualification is required and also in the voluntary, health and social interventions sectors.

Referral into programmes that provide work trials and tasters can be a safe way of enhancing work skills. The goal is to gain work-related skills or job specific skills and to do this actual work, or work tasters may be arranged. Additionally, work simulation could be arranged to gain potential skills or to renew skills in a safe and controlled environment. Sheltered work used to be common as part of industrial therapy provision, but this was shown to be less effective than open employment opportunities. Job simulation, if used, needs to be a step into the real work environment. Job simulation can be used as a therapeutic environment to practise new work skills without the risk of losing a job, which could be emotionally and financially devastating.

Managing and improving social issues for work

Housing

While housing does not necessarily seem to relate to return to work, it can have an impact on the client because having a roof over your head would be more important for most people than having a job. This is entirely reasonable, as most of us would like to know we had the security of a place to call home before considering employment. Advice on the full spectrum of housing options locally such as residential care, housing associations, council-owned houses and private rental homes are available from the local authority housing department and from independent organisations such as Citizens Advice Bureaux, some social work departments and independent providers associated with housing.

The charity Shelter (www.shelter.org.uk) provides broad advice regarding housing in the UK, taking into consideration the variation of laws and regulations that apply to each devolved country. They cover the following topics comprehensively:

- Homelessness
- Finding a home
- Paying for a home
- Renting and leasehold

- Eviction
- Repossession
- Repairs and bad conditions
- Housing issues to do with families and relationships

Other relevant organisations are the National Housing Federation (www.housing.org.uk). This organisation represents housing associations and its mission is to

'support and promote the work that housing associations do and campaign for better housing and neighbourhoods.' (www.housing.org.uk)

The Housing Corporation (www.housingcorp.gov.uk) is the national government agency that funds new affordable housing and regulates housing associations in England. The equivalent organisation in Scotland is the agency in the Scottish Executive is called Communities Scotland (www.communitiesscotland.gov.uk). The Welsh Assembly has a department responsible for housing and information (new.wales.gov.uk). In Northern Ireland housing is dealt with through the Northern Ireland Housing Executive (NIHE) (www.nihe.gov.uk).

Family responsibilities

Someone who has a caring role in a family, either for a child or an adult, may need advice about local services such as childcare, adult day care and respite care to help a family with caring. A family may need advice about funding options that are available for these services. Sure Start (www.surestart.gov.uk) is the government programme to help children and families and it offers a wide range of information about families and childcare. The Government website (www.direct.gov.uk) has a specific section about caring for someone while working. Your local authority social services department will be able to advise about help that may be available in your area and they will be able to let you know if you or your client is eligible to receive respite care or financial help with caring.

Again this is not necessarily seen as vocational rehabilitation, but unless someone can feel safe to leave a loved one they care for, it is likely to remain an obstacle to them returning to work.

Litigation and claims

Some clients will be part of a litigation claim having been in an accident at work, in a motor vehicle or in a public place. Insurance companies and solicitors can advise about a claim and Citizens Advices Bureaux can also provide advice. It is useful to have an awareness of the processes involved in a litigation case, even if you are not involved directly. The whole process is usually emotionally draining for the client and can involve a busy schedule of visiting experts to obtain reports for the courts, as well as answering lots of correspondence associated with it. As well as the claim occurring in a person's life they may also be adjusting to a new lifestyle due to impairments or disabilities and all the emotional and functional difficulties that may be apparent. The person may also be continuing with active rehabilitation and medical care, so it is a very busy time.

A document produced by the Association of Personal Injury Lawyers (2004) called *Best Practice Guide on Rehabilitation* is useful in orientating oneself to the area of rehabilitation associated with claims. It focuses on a voluntary rehabilitation code that was developed in 1999 between insurers and claimant solicitors. The rehabilitation code was developed to promote co-operation between parties involved in the rehabilitation process, which also pertains to vocational rehabilitation and return to work.

Settlement of a claim can help to bring to an end a stressful and busy period of a person's life. Being part of a litigation process can take up much time and energy and having this come to an end can mean the start of new decisions about working.

Finances

Benefits advice and financial advice are crucial to making informed decisions about the impact of starting work or retiring from work. Certain rules will need to be adhered to if a client is currently claiming benefits and wants to try out work but not lose some entitlement to the benefits. The family as a whole may need advice on claiming benefits and the effect of someone within the family unit starting work again or retiring from working. Advice from Jobcentre Plus or Citizens Advice Bureaux can be essential in making choices. Particular advice on the options will not be given here as the rules around benefits change and as such it is more appropriate to obtain up-to-date information locally.

Retirement on ill-health grounds needs to be examined carefully by an individual to make sound choices, as this can often affect an individual's pension. Often occupational health and human resources are involved in making this decision together with advocacy from the trades union or a solicitor. The client may need to seek independent financial advice to manage their pension plan and other financial policies they may have, such as income protection or policies that insure against permanent disability. The financial advice should come from a suitably qualified person who is working under the rules of the Financial Services Authority (FSA).

Being out of work can be a catalyst for getting into debt and debt counselling is a specialised area of welfare rights advice. Assisting someone to overcome his or her worries about debt can take a huge weight off their mind. Citizens Advice Bureaux often have a specialist trained in debt counselling and the National Debt Line (www.nationaldebtline.co.uk) can also offer advice that is relevant to England, Scotland and Wales.

Community access

Advice on how to access community services and facilities can help to reduce a person's social isolation. Advice to community services including shops is equally important under the Disability Discrimination Act 1995. Accessibility can be in the form of mobile services such as banking, domiciliary services such as home helps and online services such as grocery shopping. The organisation DisabledGo (www.disabledgo.info) provides a free online database of venues and services around the UK that have appropriate access to disabled people. They say:

> 'DisabledGo access guides to goods and services have been specially designed to answer the everyday questions of disabled people, their assistants, carers, family and friends. Our aim is to use access information to empower people to enjoy their communities and make their contribution.' (www.disabledgo.info)

The Disabled Persons Transport Advisory Committee (DPTAC) is an independent body set up by Government in the 1980s to provide advice about the transport needs and the access needs of disabled people. DPTAC (www.dptac.gov.uk) covers the whole of the UK.

Transport and mobility

Advice about accessibility of public transport can facilitate looking at how someone would get to and from work independently. Different types of public transport are working towards disabled access, such as the low-entry buses that are easier for wheelchairs to roll onto, or personal assistance that is available at most railway stations. This information is available from the door-to-door programme at DPTAC.

Training to use public transport can also be an important element to someone's rehabilitation, especially if they have difficulties remembering when to alight.

Advice also needs to be given about funding for public transport. There is usually a package of discounts available if transport is used regularly, and railcards that provide discounted train fares.

Drivers may need specialist advice regarding vehicle adaptations and some driving lessons or advice. This would normally involve advice about informing DVLA and the motor insurance company about changes in function and major health changes. For instance, there are particular rules regarding driving following certain surgical procedures or illnesses.

Advice about mobility-related benefits would be required as well as how these can be used in the Motability scheme (www.motability.co.uk) that helps people on mobility benefits afford a vehicle. Motability describe their services as having:

> 'overall responsibility for the Motability Scheme; determining its policy and strategic direction, overseeing the performance of the service providers who operate the Scheme under contract to Motability, and providing technical services to customers and the adaptation and conversion industry. The Motability Car Schemes are administered on a contract basis by Motability Operations, a not-for-profit private company owned by the major banks. The Wheelchair and Scooter Schemes are operated by route2mobility, a limited company, under contract to Motability.'

Accessibility to parking for disabled drivers is important and advice is available on car parks and the Blue Badge Scheme from the Direct.gov website (www.direct.gov.uk).

Specific advice for disabled motorcyclists can be found through the National Association for Bikers with a Disability (NABD) and advice for disabled motorists can be found through the newly merged organisation Mobilise.

Career choice and skills

Government departments

All the UK Government departments that are associated with helping adults to choose work, become skilled in work and achieving potential to learn further are committed to the concept of lifelong learning. This is the concept that 'It's never too soon or too late for learning', a philosophy that has taken root in a whole host of different organisations. Lifelong learning is attitudinal – one can and should be open to new ideas, decisions, skills or behaviours. Lifelong learning sees citizens provided with learning opportunities at all ages and in numerous contexts: at work, at home and through leisure activities, not just through formal institutions.

Directgov (www.direct.gov.uk) has a 'jobs and careers' search facility with more than 800 career profiles. Details of the careers as well as the training requirements, and the personal attributes that might be helpful in a particular career are explained. Voluntary work is also explained and it is possible to search for local opportunities through this website. Voluntary work can be used to help with career decision making before embarking on a particular training route.

The Department for Education and Skills (DfES) is the English Government department that has the role of

> 'creating opportunity, releasing potential and achieving excellence for all.' (www.dfes.gov.uk)

In 2004, DfES published the *Five Year Strategy for Children and Learners* in which there is a section targeted at adult skills. The goal for adult skills encompasses the ideals that employers should be able to recruit people with the right skills, and that individuals should be able to get the training and skills they need for employment and development (DfES 2004).

The Scottish Executive Department of Enterprise, Training and Lifelong Learning (www.scotland.gov.uk) has the role of

> 'supporting business, encouraging enterprise, improving skills and employability.' (www.scotland.gov.uk)

The topic of education and training within this department has a section that addresses careers as well as lifelong learning opportunities.

In the Welsh Assembly (new.wales.gov.uk), the Department for Education, Lifelong Learning and Skills (DELLS) has a role of improving children's services, education and training provision to secure better outcomes for learners (including adult learners), business, and employers.

The Northern Ireland Office has the Department for Employment and Learning (www.delni.gov.uk) whose role it is to promote learning and skills to prepare people for work and to support the economy.

Learning and skills authorities

Careers choice and education are closely connected and Learning Skills Council for England (LSC) demonstrates this in its statement:

> 'We are responsible for planning and funding high-quality vocational education and training for everyone.' (LSC website 2006)

The governments of the UK have developed skills training for individuals and employers. Sometimes these are contracted out to local providers or national providers. In March 2005 DfES in England published a White Paper called *Skills: Getting On In Business, Getting On At Work* that sets out the Department's strategy for making sure that employers have the correct skills to support the success of their businesses and sets out how individuals can gain the skills they need to be employable (DfES website 2006).

The way the training is arranged is quite similar in each country, but the schemes and programmes have different names. If you or your client want to explore these opportunities, go to the appropriate website to start your search.

The LSC has brought together

> 'the skills of the Training and Enterprise Councils and the Further Education Funding Council to work with partners, employers, learning providers, community groups and individuals to develop and implement strategies that meet the Government's aims set out in the "Learning to Succeed" White Paper.'

The equivalent organisations in Scotland are Scottish Enterprise and Highlands and Islands Enterprise (www.hie.co.uk and www.scottish-enterprise.com). Among their roles as the economic development agencies for Scotland are to develop skills in businesses, provide business support services, and deliver training and learning programmes (HIE and Scottish Enterprise websites 2006). In Wales this service is provided through the Education and Skills Department of the Welsh Assembly and details are available on their website describing the schemes available in Wales. In Northern Ireland the Department for Employment and Learning describes the skills and training opportunities to individuals and employers on their website.

Further education

Further education (FE) is that which occurs after age 16 and is not taught in a school, and *higher education* leads to a degree or higher degree usually in a university. Further education establishments are independently run and include education programmes in:

- Work-related courses such as those which lead to National or Scottish Vocational Qualifications (NVQs or SVQs), general NVQs and Business & Technology Education Council (BTEC) national diplomas
- Academic courses up to A-level standard
- Courses which are levels 1–6 on Scottish Credit and Qualifications Framework
- Basic skills courses, such as literacy and numeracy
- Courses that do not lead to a formal qualification, such as independent living skills courses
- Foundation courses that are not an integral part of a degree course
- Continuing or adult education courses
                (Skill: National Bureau for Students with Disabilities website 2004)

Within the range of FE colleges are some specialist colleges that have courses developed especially for disabled students. Funding for FE colleges is complex and can require strands of funding from several different statutory and non-statutory organisations. The charity Skill (www.skill.org.uk) can provide advice and information on aspects of funding as well as comprehensive information about learning and employment.

Online learning is available through Learndirect (www.learndirect.co.uk), which aims to:

- Reach those with few or no skills and qualifications who are unlikely to participate in traditional forms of learning
- Equip people with the skills they need for employability, thereby strengthening the skills of the workforce and increasing productivity
- Deliver innovatively through the use of new technologies

Learndirect has over 2000 online learning centres around England, Wales and Northern Ireland. Scotland has its own organisation called Learndirect Scotland (www.learndirectscotland.com).

Teaching is provided in many different locations using different modalities and with a range of qualified teachers and teaching staff who may be experts in their field but not necessarily qualified teachers – depending on the particular course that is chosen. Skills for life courses are designed to improve literacy and numeracy and some life skills and skills for work are courses designed to look at the basic skills required in open employment.

Specific information regarding lifelong education providers is available at Lifelong Learning UK (www.lifelonglearninguk.org) an organisation that is a registered charity; and the Sector Skills Council responsible for the professional development of all those working in lifelong learning. These sectors are divided into:

- Community learning and development
- Further education

- Higher education
- Libraries, archives and information services
- Work-based learning

The community-based learning and development sector aims to help individuals to develop greater self-confidence and to influence the quality of life in their community.

'Community leaders and employers make an important contribution to social cohesion and civic renewal across the UK.' (www.lifelonglearninguk.org)

Lifelong Learning UK describe work-based learning as covering

'a broad range of activity, including programmes undertaken by commercial and voluntary sector providers funded under contract to government departments and agencies, as well as a significant amount of privately funded independent and in-company training.' (www.lifelonglearninguk.org)

Trades unions

The Trades Union Congress (TUC) has developed a website called unionlearn (www.unionlearn.org.uk) to help unions spread the lifelong learning message to union members. Unionlearn was previously known as Union Academy. One of the aims for unionlearn is to

'broker learning opportunities for their members, running phone and online advice services, securing the best courses to meet learners' needs.' (www.unionlearn.org.uk)

It provides a valuable information, advice and guidance facility where union members can get individual help related to their own learning. The other important scheme relevant for vocational rehabilitation is the skills for life service where basic life skills related to reading, writing, maths and speaking English are highlighted.

The TUC and individual unions such as Unison or Amicus will also give support to their members who are struggling with issues around exploring redeployment or ill-health retirement. They will be a source of knowledge or workers' rights and legal rights for employees. Information about unions in the UK is available on the TUC website.

Department of Work and Pensions (DWP)

Jobcentre Plus (JCP) can help people to look at returning to work and the Jobcentre Personal Advisors can help to this end by advising on options and schemes available to support people to return to work. The incapacity benefit personal advisors help people who claim this benefit and they often work in co-operation with the Disability Employment Service, which is also part of JCP. If someone has a disability or a health condition that is causing barriers to return to work the Disability Employment Advisor (DEA) may get involved to offer some specialised schemes within DWP. The DEA can also help people who are struggling at work because of their disability or health condition and advise on training opportunities, job retention and job searching. The DEA can offer some schemes in certain circumstances – the qualifying criteria need to be checked with the local advisor. The schemes it currently offers (March 2007) involve:

- An employment assessment that may be carried out initially by the DEA and if needs be an enhanced assessment will be carried out by experts with relevant training such as an occupational psychologist. This helps to identify what training would be suitable and what kind of work might be suitable for an individual.
- Preparing individuals for work through a structured preparation programme. The needs of the individual are identified through the employment assessment. This scheme is provided by contracted services, is individualised and can last a few days or weeks on a part-time or full-time basis.
- Schemes to introduce a client to a new job while providing the employer with a financial grant for a limited period. This is designed to lessen the pressure to succeed.
- Job brokering under the New Deal for Disabled People where brokers prepare people for finding jobs and in job searching and facilitating interviews.
- A job matching service and the DEA can liaise with employers on the disabled person's behalf.
- Information on which local employers are recognised by the disability 'two ticks' symbol.
- Referral to specialist employment programmes such as the WORKSTEP programme. This is a scheme to help people with more complex obstacles to return to work and job retention. This scheme is provided by contracted services that are often registered charities or voluntary organisations. The provider introduces the client to the employer, supports both parties and draws up a development plan for skills and personal development.
- Referral to the Access to Work service to provide help to the client during interviews, such as a communicator support. Other in-work support is also available and will be touched on later in this chapter.

(Directgov website 2006 and Lampdirect website 2006)

The career guidance sector

The Institute of Career Guidance (ICG) defines career guidance as

> *'services and activities intended to assist individuals of any age and at any point throughout their lives, to make educational, training and occupational choices and to manage their careers. Such services may be found in schools, universities*

and colleges, in training institutions, in public employment services, in the work-place, in the voluntary or community sector and in the private sector. The activities may take place on an individual or group basis and may be face-face or at a distance.' (www.icg-uk.org)

The ICG explains that the career guidance sector can have a very wide remit to help people and this could include information and education about careers and jobs, assessment tools, career counselling, education to develop individuals' personal skills, job tasters, job searching and transition into work. In the UK there is some statutory provision of career guidance for young people and there are some Learning Skills Council-funded schemes that provide career guidance. Career guidance is also provided in the voluntary, independent and the charity sectors.

The ICG has a Register of Guidance Practitioners who have demonstrated certain levels of qualifications and experience.

Learndirect has an advice service that

'provides information, advice and guidance to support adults in making appro-priate decisions on a full range of learning and work opportunities.'

Learndirect explains that the service is free to all adults in England, Wales and Northern Ireland, that it is a confidential and impartial service and is delivered by competent and qualified helpline staff. Learndirect also offers a personalised careers advice and guidance to people who:

● Have yet to receive a full level 3 qualification
● Are returning to work
● Have been made redundant or are facing redundancy

(Learndirect website 2006)

Careers advice is also available in most schools, colleges and universities and Connexions and contacts can be seen in Table 4.6.

Independent, voluntary and charity sector providers

Individual practitioners who may or may not hold any qualification or experience in career guidance may be situated in a wide range of organisations throughout these sectors. Many people believe it is all right to give someone some career advice, and it may well be all right as long as it does not have a negative impact on the person. But, for instance, if your career advice led to someone taking a job that then exacerbated an illness you were not aware of, or led to someone having an accident because they could not read safety notices, that well-meaning advice may not be deemed so useful. While it may not be necessary to professionalise the ser-vice of giving career advice to the extent that it reduces the number of potential practitioners, it should be recognised that a client can receive 'a bit of advice' as carefully considered recommendations.

Table 4.6 Providers of career services.

Provider type	How to find them
Graduate Prospects is the UK's official graduate careers support service	www.prospects.ac.uk
The National Council for Workforce Education is a private, non-profit, professional organisation committed to promoting excellence and growth in workforce education at the post-secondary level	www.ncwe.org
Connexions provides confidential advice, support and information for 13–19 year olds – including careers advice. The website connexions-direct has a area called disability content that relates to choices young people are faced with and advice relating to these choices	www.connexions-direct.com
Career Wales is a guidance service for all ages	www.careerswales.com
Careers Scotland provide services, information and support to: individuals at all ages and stages of career planning people helping others with career planning employers wanting to maintain a productive workforce	www.careers-scotland.org.uk
Northern Ireland Careers Service. All-age career guidance service in Northern Ireland	www.careersserviceni.com
CRAC (Careers Research and Advisory Centre) is an independent educational charity aiming to advance the education of the public, and young persons in particular, in lifelong career-related learning for all	www.crac.org.uk
CASCAiD have a range of products online and available on discs. Examples of these are Adult Directions and Careers Match	www.cascaid.co.uk

There is seemingly a plethora of organisations that provide career advice in the UK. Googling 'career advice UK' brought up nearly 94.5 million possible hits! But with regards to vocational rehabilitation, the organisations that are most likely to provide careers guidance are those that also provide related services such as job searching and work preparation, work support services. For example, the Shaw Trust (www.shaw-trust.org.uk) and Employment Opportunities for Disabled People (www.opportunities.org.uk) are two of a number of organisations providing this kind of support. Some case managers may have some training in career guidance and this may be additional skill to offer clients. Some occupational psychologists may offer career guidance as part of their remit and you will be able to locate these people in the same way as indicated in Table 4.3.

Job and recruitment agencies

Agencies that specialise in locating jobs for people are abundant. How you access this information is also wide ranging. You might telephone agencies to search for a job; you might look in local newspapers, or the Yellow Pages. The high street Jobcentre Plus is an obvious choice when looking at agencies and it should also be able to signpost to the New Deal for Disabled People Job Brokers in a locality. The jobs it advertises are also available as an online search at www.jobcentreplus.gov.uk.

The Recruitment and Employment Confederation (REC) (www.rec.uk.com) is the organisation that represents this industry. Members have to meet certain qualifications and standards as well as following a code of good practice. REC also provides training to the recruitment industry with industry specific qualifications. With regards to disabled people's needs and rights, the REC provides advice and information as part of its diversity policy.

One helpful website that is a database for many agencies in this business is called Agency Central (www.agencycentral.co.uk). This website allows both employers and potential employees to search for vacancies according to type of work, geographical location and income. The database holds information regarding agencies and other websites that may specialise in a particular line of work. One particularly useful aspect is the website's ability to list recruitment agencies in a particular town, which is very handy if you are a practitioner who works across a large geographical area. Another useful aspect is the ability to search for particular job types in a town. So if you needed to see the availability of heavy goods vehicle (HGV) driving jobs in Derby you would be able to bring up an appropriate list.

Another database-styled website is youreable (www.youreable.com), which is designed for disabled people. It provides information on products and services and covers a wide range of life issues with work being one of those. The site advertises vacancies as well as providing links to other websites.

Barrierfree-recruitment.com (www.barrierfree-recruitment.com) describes itself as an interactive demonstration of what an organisation needs to do to achieve barrier-free e-recruitment for everyone. The website has been developed by the Employers' Forum on Disability with the support of the London Development Agency. It demonstrates and provides information on best practice when using e-recruitment as a medium for obtaining new employees. The jobs advertised on the website are for demonstration only, they are not real vacancies.

Whichever website you use, it may be more advantageous in the first instance to use a large database-styled website that holds information about lots of different agencies. Then it is possible to refine one's search to a locality and be aware of many of the local agencies and finally refine the search gain to one individual agency.

Job brokers are organisations that can help locate appropriate job vacancies in open employment and support people with health conditions and disabilities move into work – both before attaining a job and afterwards for a limited period of time. The New Deal for Disabled People (NDDP) is a Government employment programme and part of the Welfare to Work Strategy and it is this programme that enables a UK wide network of job brokers. The job brokers are organisations that are typically not-for-profit companies based on social firms ideals or voluntary organisations or charities. Recent qualitative research through the

Department for Work and Pensions has sought to evaluate the wide variety of services provided by job brokers (Davis et al. 2006). New Deal for Disabled People job brokers can be found on a database called job broker search (www.jobbrokersearch.gov.uk) which has details of all the job brokers in England, Scotland and Wales. The site allows you view the contact details and brief information on the services that are afforded by a provider. In Northern Ireland the place to get contact details of the job brokers is on the Department for Employment and Learning (www.delni.gov.uk). Information regarding eligibility can be sought through Directgov or the NDDP website (http://nddp.com).

With all the potential services in NDDP job brokering, checking if the provider has been accredited with the Matrix Standard can assist customers in discerning quality in services.

> 'The Matrix Standard is the unique quality framework for the effective delivery of information, advice and/or guidance on learning and work.'
> (www.matrixstandard.com)

The Matrix Standard has replaced the original National Quality Standards for Learning and Work, which were introduced to ensure that the information, advice and guidance services funded by the Government were of a high quality. The Matrix Standard has eight elements, four focused on service delivery and four focused on management of a service (www.matrixstandard.com).

Producers of materials

This sector also includes those businesses and organisations that develop career and training materials suitable to help disabled people to get into or return to work. These materials may be self-administered in a booklet form or online, they may require a trained practitioner to administer them such as a psychometric test or they may be explorative materials to learn about careers and jobs. Many companies produce tools, one of them being CASCAiD, a Loughborough University company which utilises the university expertise to develop products. CASCAiD provide training and technical help for the products they sell. The products have the capability to capture health needs of clients, adding these in to the equation in the process of careers searching.

Self-employment

Making the decision about whether to embark on self-employment can be an important one to consider for some clients. There may be all sorts of reasons why someone may want or need to contemplate working in this way. Self-employment is not necessarily the easy option to afford a good income or the chance to work whenever wanted. Being self-employed will mean no paid holidays or bank holidays, no paid sick leave, no union support, often long hours and total responsibility for the business. However, some people will thrive on being their own boss and being in control of their working life. If working in a large organisation does not suit your client, and if taking the initiative is exciting to them, then being self-employed could be the answer.

Support in starting your business and ongoing support for an established business is available in the UK through the following organisations:

Business Link (www.businesslink.gov.uk): primarily funded by the Department of Trade and Industry, supported by a number of other Government departments, agencies and local authorities. It provides information, advice and support needed to start, maintain and grow a business. Business Link is part of the Government's campaign to promote enterprise and to make the UK the best place in the world to start and grow a business and the advice is available locally (Business Link website 2006). The equivalent organisation in Scotland is Business Gateway (www.bgateway.com) and in Wales it is Business Eye (www.businesseye.org.uk). In Northern Ireland, the organisation is Invest NI (www.investni.com).

HM Revenue and Customs (www.hmrc.gov.uk): The tax office also provides support and advice for people setting up in self-employment and business. It primarily provides information regarding the tax that will need to be paid and how the Inland Revenue determines whether a person is actually deemed self-employed or employed. It also provides other more general information regarding considerations for starting up.

Jobcentre Plus (www.jobcentreplus.gov.uk): The role that Jobcentre Plus has with people who are considering becoming self-employed is to advise individuals regarding their benefits and how these might alter with the status change.

In Biz (www.inbiz.co.uk): Promotes, develops and supports individual and group enterprise and initiative amongst all sectors of the community. This organisation provides free advice and training in setting up a business. Eligibility is through particular benefits with incapacity benefit currently being one of those. In Biz will help people work through business ideas, develop business plans through to supporting after launching a business. There is coverage over many parts of the UK.

Prince's Trust (www.princes-trust.org.uk): The Prince's Trust is a charity that works to help young people between 14 and 30 years old to overcome barriers and, 'get their lives working' (Prince's Trust website 2006). The charity provides financial assistance, training and mentoring to young disadvantaged people. It has a young persons' business start-up scheme to help young entrepreneurs aged 18 to 30.

British Chambers of Commerce (www.chamberonline.co.uk)

'The British Chambers of Commerce (BCC) is a non-political, non-profit making organisation, owned and directed by its members, democratically accountable to over 135 000 individual businesses of all sizes and sectors throughout the UK. It covers all the local Chambers of Commerce.' (BCC website 2006)

The local Chamber of Commerce can, once one is a member, provide business advice, networking and training opportunities. There is often a centre where businessmen and businesswomen can meet and where resources are available. Local Chambers of Commerce can be found in the telephone directory and through the BCC website.

Federation of Small Businesses (www.fsb.org.uk): The Federation of Small Businesses (FSB) is a non-profit-making organisation supported solely by members' subscriptions and donations. It is a non-party-political lobbying group continually campaigning for the rights of the small business. Local chambers can be found in the telephone directory and the BCC website. For people starting up a business, FSB provide support and advice related to business planning, financial forecasting, tax, legislation appropriate to sole traders and small businesses and further business advice.

Types of interventions related to career choice and skills

The mind map in Figure 4.3 showed how I see vocational rehabilitation in the UK. The category of choosing work would be the appropriate place for career guidance and in choosing work the interventions could be subdivided into vocational profiling, interviews, obtaining an offer of work and into acceptance of a work offer. Figure 4.5 now expands the second part of the mind map by suggesting in more detail the interventions that one might expect to find in choosing work, which tend to fall under career guidance and support.

Vocational profiling

All supported employment services should focus on individual choice and accurate information on jobs and the support options that are available. These give the individual the power to make informed decisions and have responsibility to accomplish goals (Leach 2002). Providing information in the correct medium for the client is a consideration, as learning occurs in different modes. Information should be available in text versions (or Braille), photos, video, and multimedia on a computer, through signing and through real-life experiences. According to the Institute of Careers Guidance careers guidance involves helping people to:

- Understand themselves, including assessing their own achievements, abilities and interests
- Investigate learning and work opportunities
- Evaluate the options open to them and decide upon the action needed
- Implement their plans for learning and work

(Institute of Careers Guidance website 2006)

Undertaking these tasks requires some depth of understanding about careers theories and the way in which people undertake career planning, career exploration, career decision making and transitioning into work again. Understanding

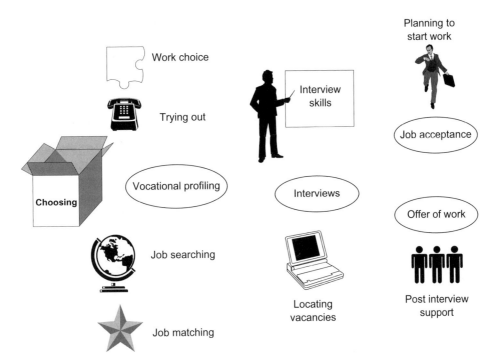

Figure 4.5 Choosing work: career guidance and support interventions.
Images from Microsoft Clip Art.

developmental career theory (Super, in Sharf 1992) social cognitive career theory (Lent et al. in Brown & Brooks 1996) and other career theories is important. Inherent in these theories is the need to gain an in-depth understanding of how your client perceives their own particular barriers to making a career choice (if indeed there are barriers) including the cognitions they express about careers, their perceived ability in career search, how persistent they are in job searching, the financial context of an individual, the environmental context of an individual and the socioeconomic patterns in a geographical area.

With this in mind, careers advice is not a task to take on lightly and it does not just require accurate information about local job availability or careers as such. In some research there is indication that being disabled can add to career indecision (Enright 1996). Being disabled may add a complexity to career beliefs (beliefs about the world of work) and career decisions for some people. Perceived career barriers may cause your client to feel anxious and unconfident in their approach to the career decision making process (Punch et al. 2005). The Joseph Rowntree Foundation agreed with differences between able-bodied and disabled people in their mid 20s and produced a report entitled *The Education and Employment of Disabled Young People: Frustrated Ambition* in 2005. It reported that:

'The scope and level of aspirations among disabled 16-year-olds were similar to those of their non-disabled counterparts . . . Disabled and non-disabled 16-year-olds expected the same level of earnings from a full-time job.'

However, by age 26 aspirations had diminished. Burchardt (2005) reported

'a widening gap between disabled and non-disabled young people as they moved into their twenties, in terms of confidence, subjective well-being and belief in their ability to shape their own future.' (Joseph Rowntree Foundation website 2006)

This seems to suggest that more should be done to narrow this gap – the vice chairperson of the National Association for Paediatric Occupational Therapists indicated in an interview with *Therapy Weekly* in December 2005 that therapists should become involved with career advice and career counselling with their clients who are in years 7 and 8 at school (Arnold 2005). Enright (1996) suggests that one way this can be achieved is for practitioners to assess how a disability may have shaped a person's self-concept and the perception that he or she has on their abilities in relation to career goals.

However, in another study it was shown that disabled people do not necessarily differ from able-bodied peers, in their career thoughts at least (Strauser et al. 2002). The term 'career thoughts' refers to those misconceptions about careers and career planning and dysfunctional thinking in career problem solving. The authors suggested that rehabilitation practitioners should not assume that disabled people have higher than usual levels of dysfunctional career thoughts. They urged practitioners to analyse each client's career thoughts to determine implications for career development and vocational rehabilitation (Strauser et al. 2002).

Vinokur et al. (2000) explain that:

'Knowledge of the psychological characteristics or vulnerabilities that impede successful re-entry into the workforce is essential for designing social interventions that aim at enhancing marketability and job search skills.'

Punch et al. (2005) indicate when talking about adolescents who are hard-of-hearing that it is important for these young people to engage in careful career exploration and planning to minimise the potential disadvantages of environmental and attitudinal barriers. Using cognitive behavioural techniques can be one way of challenging unhelpful beliefs and attitudes generally about 'suitable' career decisions for disabled people. With regard to vocational rehabilitation in the UK, it would seem pertinent to forge alliances between career guidance specialists, vocational rehabilitation specialists and service users in developing appropriate and individualised career advice.

Career search

This element is concerned with knowledge about the world of work and the wide variety of careers that are available in the 21st century. Career indecision may occur as a result of a lack of knowledge of the world of work, but this might not necessarily be construed as negative. If your client has a limited understanding of the world of work and the opportunities therein, indecision can allow a time of exploration. This in turn, according to Enright (1996) can enhance a person's confidence and belief (self-efficacy) in their ability to choose a suitable career and job.

Resources depicting careers and jobs and what they actually entail as far as day-to-day tasks will be required in different media. Creating understanding regarding the world of work may make it clearer to your client what goals they want to strive for. The practitioner offering the guidance will not necessarily be familiar with all jobs that are in existence, but they should be aware of job databases where this information is stored. One such resource of occupational information is a United States official website called Occupational Information Network (www.onetcenter.org).

In social cognitive career theory, goals are a significant predictor of career development and career behaviours (planning and exploration, for instance). The goal is used to guide a client's behaviour towards achieving an outcome and this is usually linked to what the expected outcome is believed to be. How persistent your client is in working towards the goal will be determined partly through self-efficacy, locus of control and partly through complex internal and external barriers (Brown & Brooks 1996; Strauser 2002; Punch et al. 2005).

Career counselling

In this context counselling is referring to the facilitative approach in which practitioners engage with their clients during the process of choosing work and re-employment. Practitioners should have counselling skills as part of their repertoire and advanced skills in cognitive behavioural techniques, or other related skills such as family therapy will be of benefit. Career counselling is concerned with identifying career alternatives and developing strategies to reach the goal. Career counselling may not be appropriate for everyone and career guidance may suffice but some clients will need the time to have a deeper exploration of their beliefs and feelings (self-awareness) and the barriers and opportunities that affect them in career decision making. In vocational rehabilitation there should be equal emphasis on issues relating to disability and or health issues that are affecting the client's career choices.

Career counselling is not about pursuing career aspirations that will never be possible to achieve, but it is concerned with opening a client's awareness to the possibility of valued work that is achievable. The client who wants to work as a lawyer to pursue justice as a cause may not in fact be aware of all the other career avenues that might achieve the underlying personal aspiration. A plumber with a painful back may feel he or she is now unsuitable for the job but with careful analysis of the situation by the career counsellor it may emerge that plumbing remains a feasible option if some alterations to routines and working hours are made.

The individual practitioner will tend to use their own philosophical background to construct the intervention with their client. This may be based on their profession's theories or other profession's theories. One such theory is Hershenson's theory of work adjustment (Strauser et al. 2002) and for which a detailed description of the theory can be sought from Hershenson (1996).

In essence, though, the theory has been constructed with disabled people in mind, and to address both congenital and acquired disabilities on career development, Strauser et al. (2002) explain that interventions in vocational rehabilitation and career counselling that focus on developing work competencies (work habits, physical and mental skills and work-related interpersonal skills) may have some effect on work personality (self-concept as a worker, systems for motivation for work and work-related needs and values). Strauser et al. also reflect that the positive outcome of improved work personality is that:

> *'Individuals with well developed work personality report higher levels of job readiness self-efficacy and more internalised work locus of control.'*

Further, self-efficacy in job readiness is important because the client who believes that he or she will be successful in job searching is more likely to obtain employment. It seems vital that in a vocational rehabilitation programme, career guidance and counselling sit alongside the other interventions that are offered, such as cognitive behavioural therapy or work hardening.

Figure 2.3 showed a career decision making process that a career counsellor may work through to help a client re-enter work. No one approach will suit every client but the key asset to each career counselling programme is the active engagement of the client and collaborative working to achieve the client's goals.

Financial advice
Part of the decision making process for an individual will involve weighing up the financial implications for returning to work or staying on benefits, for taking a promotion or staying put or for entering voluntary work. In nearly every decision that is made regarding work there is likely to be an element that involves finances. The decisions may not be as straightforward as should I come off benefits or not? They may involve complex situations to do with mortgage repayments, insurance policies or children's childcare costs. Decisions about working part-time versus full-time, overtime payments and bonus payments are really beneficial and are also financially related. Whatever the questions are, the answers that are provided to your client must be accurate. Questions about how employment arrangements will affect an individual's tax are also a consideration for many people and advice can be sought through the local tax office. Unless you are qualified to give advice about benefits, tax or financial information you need to refer this task to a suitably qualified practitioner. Financial advice is bound by rules from the Financial Services Authority and this should be borne in mind if you recommend that your clients seek financial advice.

Legal and employment rights advice
Clients should be aware of their rights within an employment situation, and accurate and pertinent information needs to be communicated in a way that will be

understood by the client. It is highly unlikely that the majority of the population would be able to clearly decipher legal documents and law. Your client may have a disability and be covered by the Disability Discrimination Act (DDA) 1995 and as such you may need to inform him or her and the potential employer of the basics of this Act. More in-depth information may need to be provided by a specialist in employment law, including the ramifications of the DDA.

Specialist advisors will be able to give advice at Citizens Advice Bureaux and the trades unions may also be able to give help. In the context of career decision making, the trades union may be involved in giving advice about the rights of its members with regards to ill-health retirement and helping the employee to contribute to the decisions taken by the employer. Likewise, the union may provide advice about other in-house job opportunities and employment rights associated with redeployment or the DDA for instance. Relevant legislation will include but not be limited to:

- Health and Safety at Work Act 1974
- Management of Health and Safety at Work Regulations 1999
- Disability Discrimination Act 1995
- Employment Rights Act 1996
- Employment Act 2002
- Data Protection Act 1998
- The Welfare Reform Bill (208) 2006
- The Compensation Act (October 2006)
- The Employment Equality (Age) Regulations 2006

Job tasters

If your client has not had experience in different work environments they may find it useful to try out some different jobs over a day or couple of days. *Job tasters* are useful in providing your client with tangible information about work. They are the real thing and not necessarily the ideal picture that can be interpreted from a book or even a video. They are particularly useful in providing the experiential learning that for some people will be more appropriate and create a longer lasting memory than other modes of learning. There is nothing quite like being in a work environment to get the 'feeling' of the place. All the senses are bombarded and there is social interaction with real people doing the actual job.

Job tasters can last varying amounts of time from a couple of hours to several days. They require careful planning and the client may need support before, during and afterwards to cope with the experience and to synthesise the new experience adequately. Job tasters can be viewed as part of the assessment process, but when the whole process of choosing a career and work and then searching for a job is such a dynamic one, it is difficult to pinpoint where the assessment finishes and the intervention starts.

Essentially with any of these ways of exploring potential options with your client, the aim for the practitioner is to make it a positive experience from which the client comes away having a greater belief in their capability to do a job or type of work. This is working on your client's self-efficacy in particular tasks. Increasing your client's self-efficacy in choosing the right kind of work is thought to have better results if your client can be part of discussions about work, even better if they can see someone doing that job and better still if they can have a go at it and accomplish the task. But of course, this needs managing in the right way. The job taster may not turn out so well – but the choices for work may now be narrowed, which might be a good outcome for the client.

Your client may be quite able to go and search for the job and work they have decided upon without any assistance from anyone. If this is the case, then you may only need to point them in the direction of the newspaper or the Jobcentre. However, for many people the idea of job searching is a daunting task fraught with potential points of failure. If support is required for this process there are a number of ways this can be achieved. It is important to remember that:

'Job search is a joint outcome of the search effort of job seekers and the hiring decisions of employers.' (Vinokur et al. 2000)

Programmes are available to support your client in job searching in the form of job clubs and one-to-one guidance. Vinokur and Schul (2002) suggest that a programme for job searching can include addressing the following issues for an individual:

- Job search efficacy (belief in the ability to search for jobs)
- Job search motivation
- Mastery of searching (linked to efficacy)
- Financial strain involved with looking for work
- Job search intensity on the part of the person doing the searching
- (Symptoms for those people who are at risk of becoming or are already likely to have an exacerbation of symptoms). This has been put in parenthesis because it is not directly part of the searching process, but is related to the intensity that someone takes part.

Programmes have been developed to help people improve their persistence and skills in job searching. The programmes are based on particular theories such as the cognitive behavioural model, social learning theory, learned optimism and self-efficacy and as such they help to challenge and reassign negative thoughts and beliefs into positive ones. Researchers say this changes thoughts and behaviours, resulting in improved persistence to job searching and obtaining work.

One such programme in Australia is called the *Changing Wonky Beliefs* training, which Tony Machin and Peter Creed says strives towards

'participants learning the skills associated with the approach of flexible optimism and to be motivated to practice them in such a way as to make them habitual.' (University of Southern Queensland website 2006) (Creed et al. 1999)

Another programme is the JOBS programme for the unemployed, situated in the USA. This has been evaluated in a research paper (Vinokur et al. 2000).

Job matching

In deciding what kind of work is practical for a client to undertake, you and your client will both require an understanding of the current functional abilities as well as the aspirations concerning what they would like to be able to do in work. This information will be gained through accurate and detailed assessments as described in Chapter 2. It is important to remember that a person's functional abilities change over time and so do aspirations. And for this reason it is imperative that the practitioner does not assume that the information that was gained a number of weeks ago, remains valid.

Supports required

It is a useful exercise to check regularly with your client about the supports that would be seen as helpful in a workplace. Depending on the nature of the work and the context of the work environment, this may also change. Understanding of appropriate supports may be based on prior experiences and current needs of your client. The process to investigate support requirements is a positive one, and should not be about excluding an individual from a particular job necessarily. The exploration may involve developing a support needs checklist (Leach 2002) that can then be updated on a regular basis as needs change. For instance, a fluctuating medical condition may result in your client requiring supports intermittently. So someone with multiple sclerosis, for instance, may sometimes require some mobility support in the form of a wheelchair accessible environment or IT support for a computer in the form of voice-activated software when movement in hands may be affected. This will not always be required, but is essential information to have on a support needs checklist. An example of a support needs checklist can be seen in Table 4.7.

This checklist is something tangible to take along to interviews if this is seen as helpful, and allows the prospective employer to be aware. It can also be used with an existing employer as part of return to work planning.

Part of the exercise on job matching is liaising with workplaces to establish accurate information about the work, the workplace, the organisational structure, remuneration and duties. If your client is at the stage where they have not yet decided what it is they would feel comfortable working as, then researching several job profiles to establish if there is a potential fit will be a useful exercise.

Interviews

In the UK, employers that have the two ticks badge have shown themselves to be particularly disability-friendly, which may be useful to narrow a potential list for disabled people. Two ticks and the words 'positive about disabled people' represent the disability symbol given to employers by Jobcentre Plus, and it is displayed on job adverts and application forms. The symbol recognises employers who have agreed to make positive commitments about the employment, retention, training

Table 4.7 Example of a support needs checklist.

Need	Support required	Frequency/duration	Resources	Cost
Mobility – difficulty walking more than 100 metres	Personal assistance (walk alongside) from the car park to the office	Every relapse of symptoms Usually lasting three weeks	Colleague at work	Zero
Dexterity – difficulty co-ordinating fingers at speed	Alternative method of inputting information into the computer	Most days, but likes to use the keyboard when possible	Speech software compatible with employer's computing system	£170
	Alternative method of dialling telephone numbers	Every day	Automatic dialler	£50
Hospital appointments to attend	Time off for rehabilitation and to see the consultant	Every three months, once per week to see the physio for one hour	Sanctioned time off outside of annual and sick leave	Hourly rate while on appointments

and career development of disabled people (Direct.gov website 2006). Disability employment advisors have a list of local companies that have signed up to this symbol.

Many of the job brokers and Connexions will have a range of resources that clients can make use of to help in the search for an appropriate job, but job searching requires resources from as many different angles as possible. They include your client, their family and friends, other service providers the client may be involved with, the disability employment advisor, Jobcentre Plus, the incapacity benefit personal advisor and anyone else you can think of who may know of a vacancy that would be suitable. Resources may be in the form of training for job searching, the world of work and local opportunities. If you have already managed the previous two issues then a locality search is next on the list.

Locality-based searches of the local opportunities are essential. It is not particularly helpful to identify a career path and type of job that then does not exist in reasonable amounts locally. Locally can mean any distance that is feasible for your client to travel to routinely. So for one person locally might mean within a two-mile walk of their house and for another person it might mean within one day's travelling and could be Europe. The information about jobs can come from:

- Websites
- Newspapers
- Local small advertisements in shops
- Word of mouth
- Cold calling
- Job finding services

Jobs around the country will differ depending on the heritage of an area, the road, rail, air and sea transport links, the landscape, the population density and natural resources. This diversity should be recognised and the positive aspects of the job market built on. Just by looking in a local newspaper, the Yellow Pages or contacting the local Chamber of Commerce can help in understanding a particular location. This will be an important task to undertake if you are a practitioner who works across a wide geographical area rather than your own local patch, because you will not be so familiar with job opportunities.

Help and advice in completing application forms can be vital. I have often heard of colleagues whose clients have not before previously had any help, and have not been following the basic instructions in an application form such as 'use black ink'. Checking that spellings are correct, completing the form in pencil first, photocopying the form to practise, or completing the form on a computer can give your client the time to be satisfied with the form before sending it off.

Various organisations such as those mentioned in Table 4.6 advise on completing application forms. The Directgov website has a section that advises people on how to complete forms, write covering letters and write application letters. They have examples of adverts and job descriptions as well as examples of letters and curricula vitae (CVs). All these forms require written communication skills of a certain degree and if your client is going to call the employer to clarify points on the advert, then verbal communication will also be required. You may feel it is appropriate to prepare your client in advance to give him or her the best chance to succeed. If it is felt that reasonable adjustment is required regarding assisting someone fill out a form, it is an idea to call the employer to investigate this option further. For instance, someone who is partially sighted who would not be able to complete a standard application form in handwriting. Using constructive feedback on how application forms are perceived by the employer can be useful to make future changes. A dummy run could be arranged with a similar employer to see what feedback they would give to the client.

Interview skills

Negotiating reasonable adjustments for an interview needs to be done in plenty of time. Access to Work can accept a referral to assist in this matter and they may consider a communicator for a client or assist with travel. There is an abundance of training and books about interview skills and how to behave in an interview to give the applicant the best chance of getting a job. In vocational rehabilitation, training may also be valuable to the client to look at gaining the right skills and performing in a stressful situation. This may involve role-play, peer feedback in a group setting, video feedback of real and role-play interviews, all of which are opportunities for your client to learn about:

- Communication skills
- Social skills
- Appearance

Additional information and advice – may be required regarding:

- Financial support
- Disclosure advice

When the client has been for an interview, it should be possible to obtain some feedback from the interview or interview panel. The client would be encouraged to receive this feedback and then to be supported and encouraged to make the next step, which might be attending another interview or deciding whether or not to accept the post after all. Making that decision may have to be done in a short space of time. Most employers have not got time to wait for days and days – they need to know as quickly as possible – so if your client says no thank you, they can move on to the next best candidate. Supporting your client to make an informed choice will be an important role. If your client has used all their inner resources to get to the interview and perform, they also need to be ready to make decisions about the job acceptance. There may be reasons why they feel they need to back down and say no thank you to an offer, and this may be down to anxiety about the unknown or the sudden responsibility of a new job, or it may mean having to move house, which involves the children moving schools. The list is endless, but not insurmountable. Personally speaking, I would want to go through the, 'if you are accepted in this post, will you take the job?' questioning prior to the interview rather than afterwards, to address the potential issues while there is less pressure to accept because the job has been offered.

Offer of work and job acceptance

Once your client has accepted a position with an existing employer or a new employer, then that employer puts in place their own procedures to formally engage the interviewee. This will usually entail a formal letter of acceptance, though not always, that details the terms and conditions of the employment, a potential start date and possibly a health questionnaire or a meeting with occupational health. Some new employees will need to have a Criminal Records Bureau (CRB) check carried out, and this can delay the start of a new employment period by some weeks.

You may want to talk to your client about disclosing their disability or health condition and the benefits of doing this and the possible risks associated with disclosure. There are no hard and fast rules to dictate when someone should disclose a disability. But the general advice is that:

- There is no obligation for an employer to make a reasonable adjustment where they do not know, or could not reasonably be expected to know, that you would need any adjustments – so informing a potential employer could be helpful in the long run. Employers could have grounds for dismissal if a disability is not disclosed. If a client has signed a form to say that they do not have a disability and later this is found out to be untrue there could be repercussions.
- Some people feel safer disclosing to an employer who has publicly made a commitment to employing disabled people and has the two ticks symbol or is recognised by the Disability Standard 2007 from the Employers' Forum on Disability. If a person meets the minimum criteria of the person specification in a job, the 'two ticks' symbol means they are guaranteed a job interview.
- If someone doesn't declare a disability, an employment tribunal might decide that the employer was justified in failing to make adjustments. On the other hand, it could also decide that that the employer could reasonably be expected to know about the employee's disability even if it had not been declared.
- In an interview, questions regarding disabilities on an application form or in an interview can be answered in a straightforward way, describing how the disability may have no effect on the person's capability to do the job. Focusing on abilities and requirements for the job is a more positive way forward. Being disabled may add valuable experience and skills to certain jobs and this can be a valuable reason to disclose.
- Many people are uneducated about disability and are unnecessarily frightened by the thought of certain health conditions and they may make assumptions about employing a disabled person.

Information obtained from Direct.gov, RNIB (www.rnib.org.uk), diversity.monster (www.diversity.monster.co.uk) and Employers' Forum on Disability websites 2006

Planning to start work may mean some change in routines, especially if your client has been off work for any length of time. Family will need to get used to changes, too. Trying to fit in work along with a busy life outside work can seem impossible for some clients. If your client has been in the habit of going to bed late and getting up late, then this habit will need to be rescheduled. It is quite likely that the change will be difficult, especially if the behaviour is entrenched, but a graded programme of change can help. The whole family's routines may need to accommodate another person getting up early to use the bathroom and have breakfast, and a generally busier home environment needs to be talked through and discussed. Eating breakfast is important to ensure sufficient calories for the morning, as is a drink to rehydrate the body. Planning which clothes will be required for the next day, whether a packed lunch is needed or sufficient cash is available to buy lunch are all important and can be done the night before. I have found that the key is not to wait until the weekend before someone starts work to implement these changes, but to start much earlier. But a job offer can sometimes galvanise people to make huge changes in their routines.

Organising how your client will get to work, which route, which bus to catch, which stop to get off at are all part of the planning to start a particular job. There may be a discounted public transport ticket that can be purchased to help with costs. Some clients will need to learn a route by repeated practice until it becomes habit to remember the route. In these cases, preparation can start and then your client will need continued support until they are independently managing the journey. Access to Work will consider referrals for assistance in getting to and from work. In the case of some health conditions that result in fatigue, it can be better to arrive at work with as much energy as possible and a taxi may be the answer. Also leaving work at the end of the day is usually tiring, and to be able to have a little extra support in conserving energy can mean that vital chores at home get done.

The extra pressures of finding a job, going for interviews and the emotional rollercoaster when accepting a job can all take their toll on your client's health. Managing symptom exacerbation through this period can be particularly important. This is an excellent time to work as a team in vocational rehabilitation, to support an individual in self-management and to succeed in their quest to make it into work.

Summary

In this section, the interventions associated with career choice and skills have been explored. The relevant providers of interventions have been described and suggestions made as to how to contact them. Interventions themselves have been organised into categories preparing for work, choosing work and engaging with work and it has been suggested that career choice and skills fits in the choosing work category.

Workplace-related interventions

Using vocational rehabilitation to help motivate your client and get him or her ready for working again can be very rewarding work. But all of this effort can come to an end if the workplace is not suitable for your client. There has to be a continuation of the vocational rehabilitation into the workplace to enable a successful return to work. This means:

- Communicating with employers and using their language (not medical language)
- Understanding their pressures and business commitments
- Addressing issues to do with the work environment itself

In Chapter 2 assessments related to the work environment were addressed and some of the elements in the workplace were explored. This section explores the providers of workplace-related interventions and advice. The practitioners who are involved and their potential roles are also addressed to help you understand the service or organisation a little more. This section will also look at the types of workplace interventions that are appropriate in vocational rehabilitation, give some descriptions of the interventions and some resource information to help further research.

Professionals and practitioners and their likely roles

Government departments

The Department for Work and Pensions is the government department under which the disability services sit. Access to Work (AtW) is part of the disability service and it functions out of the Jobcentre Plus offices around the UK. Access to Work is the service that provides practical assistance to those people struggling at work with a disability or long-term health condition. It was introduced as a new scheme in 1994. The Disability Coalition carried out a review of the AtW service in 2004 and describes the potential benefits as:

'The advice, financial assistance and practical support available to employers and disabled employees through AtW helps to ensure that employers need not be concerned about possible financial and technical issues arising from the appointment of a disabled person.'

Applying to AtW involves a self-referral by your client to your regional office in England, the office for Scotland or the office for Wales, details of which can be found on the Jobcentre website (www.jobcentreplus.gov.uk). In Northern Ireland the AtW service sits under the Department for Employment and Learning (www.delni.gov.uk) and referral to this service is through the disability employment advisor.

Jobcentre Plus explains the service:

'Access to Work is available to help overcome the problems resulting from disability. It offers practical advice and help in a flexible way that can be tailored to suit the needs of an individual in a particular job. AtW does not replace the normal responsibilities of the employer to implement Health and Safety regulations or replace the responsibilities required by the Disability Discrimination Act.' (www.jobcentreplus.gov.uk)

The costs associated with providing support should be checked with your local AtW service, but currently as a rule of thumb equipment bears a cost share with the employer and services costs are borne by AtW. The funding for the service has strict guidelines and as such the particular situation relating to your client requires individual analysis by AtW. The experience and qualifications of the staff within AtW varies and they have the capacity to use independent practitioners with particular areas of expertise to come in and provide specific assessments when required. I know of occupational therapists, physiotherapists and nurses who regularly carry out assessments on behalf of AtW.

The Health and Safety Executive (HSE) is sponsored by the DWP and is responsible for ensuring that risks to people's health and safety from work activities are properly controlled. The HSE (www.hse.gov.uk) and local government are the enforcing authorities that work in support of the Health and Safety Commission. As an organisation the HSE is responsible for looking after the major risks associated with industries that are involved with hazardous materials or dangerous environments as well as the health effects of workplaces on people. The HSE website has many sections about creating healthy workplaces – some relevant ones to vocational rehabilitation are:

Musculoskeletal disorders (MSDs). This section contains information about the annual Better Backs Campaign, back pain, the manual handling assessment (MAC) tool and guidance and research.

Risk management. This section of the website contains guidance on the Five Steps to risk assessment, examples of risk assessments, and industry-specific guidance e.g. agriculture industry.

Workplace Health Connect (www.workplacehealthconnect.co.uk). The website explains that the service is

'a free, no-obligation service set up in partnership with the Health and Safety Executive. We provide free, practical advice on workplace health and safety, working with both managers and staff.'

Healthy Working Lives (www.healthyworkinglives.com) is the equivalent programme in Scotland and was initiated before the Workplace Health Connect programme in England and Wales. It is not part of the HSE, but is placed here to show the comparative service.

Sickness absence and return to work. This section of the HSE website contains information about guidance for employers, including the Six Steps approach to managing sickness absence, guidance on legal issues and reasonable adjustments.

Human factors/ergonomics. This section has guidance on the law associated with ergonomics and research.

Stress. This section contains guidance on the stress management standards, good practice, stress survey tools, advice for individuals, research and statistics.

NHS Scotland has taken the telephone advice on health and safety and occupational health a step further and has the Centre for Healthy Working Lives, which has achieved this by bringing together Scotland's Health at Work (SHAW) and Safe and Healthy Working (SaHW) under the same umbrella (Health Scotland website, www.healthscotland.com).

Education

Further Education (FE) courses were explored on pp. 151–2. Employers may arrange day release for some part-time vocational courses. The learndirect scheme called Learning Through Work allows people to study without having to take time off from work and the employer meets some or all the course costs. Studying leads to a higher education degree, but not every university offers this scheme and information can be seen on the learndirect website (www.learndirect-ltw.co.uk). learndirect says:

> 'Customised programmes build on existing skills and knowledge and focus on work-related learning.'

The courses are individually designed from available modules and lead to a higher education qualification by planning and structuring learning around existing work commitments.

Occupational health

Occupational health services (OHS) are in existence to help employers' commitment to health and safety. They provide services to advise managers and employees to promote the highest standards of physical and psychological well-being. Unlike most other European Union countries, this service is not a legislative requirement in the UK. In a report to the House of Commons the Select Committee on Work and Pensions explained that:

> 'Provision (of OHS) is further endorsed as a key requirement of the EU Framework Directive (89/391) in which employers are required to manage

the work environment according to a set of prevention principles, together with workers or representatives and with the support of either internal or external prevention services.' (House of Commons Select Committee on Work and Pensions, 4th report 2004)

In a survey of OHS conducted by the HSE in 1992 only a third of the workforce had access to OHS and less than a third had no access to occupational health, not even first aid (Chambers et al. 2001). OHS are therefore not necessarily accessible through every employer and mostly not available in the small to medium enterprises, which is one reason for the HSE's new Workplace Health Connect service. Securing Health Together is the occupational health strategy for England, Wales and Scotland and was launched in 2000 (HSC 2000), having a 10-year vision about tackling work-related ill-health. Working for Health (www.workingforhealthni.gov.uk) is the long-term workplace health strategy for Northern Ireland and was written in 2003.

Within the UK, the type and extent of professional OHS varies from industry to industry (Chambers et al. 2001). If your client's employer does provide an OHS, it could be an in-house service or a contracted-in service and an OHS may encompass a range of practitioners as seen in Table 4.8. This is not an exhaustive list of practitioners, but perhaps the more common members of the occupational health team.

Table 4.8 Potential practitioners in OHS and their respective organisations.

Practitioner	Organisation	Website
Occupational health nurses	The Royal College of Nursing (RCN) represents nurses and nursing and the Society of Occupational Health Nursing promotes excellence in practice in the workplace and the importance of improving the working environment and the health of the working population	www.rcn.org.uk
	The Association of Occupational Health Nurse Practitioners (AOHNP) (UK) is a professional organisation for occupational health nurse practitioners. The Association was founded in 1992 to increase representation and raise the profile of occupational health nurses in the UK	www.aohnp.co.uk
Occupational health physicians	The Society of Occupational Medicine (SOM) is concerned with the protection of the health of people in the workplace, the prevention of occupational injuries and disease related environmental issues	www.som.org.uk
	The Faculty of Occupational Medicine (FOM) is a professional and academic body empowered to develop and maintain high standards of training, competence and professional integrity in occupational medicine	www.facoccmed.ac.uk

Table 4.8 *continued.*

Practitioner	Organisation	Website
	The Association of National Health Occupational Physicians (ANHOPS) provides occupational health services to NHS employers	www.anhops.com
Occupational health and safety practitioner	Professional Organisations in Occupational Safety and Health (POOSH) promotes the continuous improvement of the practice of occupational safety and health between all practitioners and agencies involved in the provision of a healthy and safe working environment	www.poosh.org
	The National Examination Board in Occupational Safety and Health (NEBOSH) is an independent awarding body for relevant training	www.nebosh.org.uk
Occupational hygienist	The British Occupational Hygiene Society (BOHS) is concerned with controlling health hazards at work	www.bohs.org
Health and safety officer	The Institution of Occupational Safety and Health (IOSH) is Europe's leading body for health and safety professionals. It is an independent and not-for-profit organisation aiming to regulate and steer the profession	www.iosh.co.uk
Physiotherapist	The Chartered Society of Physiotherapy (CSP) is the professional, educational and trade union body	www.csp.org.uk
	The Association of Chartered Physiotherapists in Occupational Health and Ergonomics (ACPOHE) is a specialist interest group recognised by the Chartered Society of Physiotherapy	www.acpohe.org.uk
Occupational therapist	The College of Occupational Therapists (COT) is the professional body for occupational therapists in the UK	www.cot.org.uk
	WORK is the College of Occupational Therapists specialist section for occupational therapists interested in work and productivity	www.cot.org.uk (specialist sections)
Psychologist	The British Psychological Society (BPS) is responsible for the professional activities of occupational psychologists	www.bps.org.uk
	The Division of Occupational Psychology (DOP) is part of the BPS and has a website called People and Organisations @ Work	www.pow-bps.com
Ergonomist	The Ergonomics Society represents ergonomists in the UK and strives to maintain professional standards	www.ergonomics.org.uk

NHS

NHS Plus is a network of occupational health services based in NHS hospitals. The network provides an occupational health service to NHS staff, and also sells services to the private sector. In some of the large trusts, the NHS occupational health departments have a wealth of experience that makes them a good source of advice and help for companies who are looking for an occupational health service (www.nhsplus.nhs.uk). The profits from the services that NHS Plus sells are reinvested into the NHS OHS.

Unions

Union representatives are important in negotiating return to work plans and in successful job retention. In one organisation there will not always be just one union representing the workforce, so it is important to establish which union (if any) your client is a current member with. With their permission, you may be able to call the union representative to discuss the planning and implementing of retention or return to work.

Some unions are very large organisations in their own right and the Trades Union Congress (TUC) has many of these unions associated with it. The TUC and the large unions provide training and publications on issues such as the Disability Discrimination Act 1995 and reasonable adjustments, which are of particular importance for some people returning to work or trying to remain in work. The representatives will be trained in understanding your client's issues and then in negotiating the best outcome with employers. If additional training is required by an employee, the unions will often have representatives specially trained in looking at a person's needs and then organising a training course to improve skills and knowledge. The unions may be able to offer diversity training to employers to create better working environments and healthier attitudes towards disabled people.

HSE, with the assistance of the TUC, has produced a leaflet designed to help trade union representatives work with their members to help prevent long-term sickness absence becoming job loss. The HSE describe six ways in prevention work:

1. Helping to identify measures to improve worker health, preventing it from worsening by work
2. Suggesting employers develop workplace plans and policies on sickness absence management
3. Helping to keep absent workers in touch with work
4. Helping employers to plan adjustments to enable return to work
5. Supporting workers to return to work
6. Helping to promote understanding of health conditions and disability in the workplace.

(HSE 2005b)

Advice/legal sector

The Citizens Advice Bureaux (CAB) has nationwide coverage and is an extremely useful organisation in providing independent advice about employer and employee rights at work and other related issues that may be pertinent in returning to work.

The Advisory, Conciliation and Arbitration Service (ACAS) is an independent organisation that aims to improve organisations and working life through improved employment relations. It was set up following the introduction of the Employment Protection Act 1975, bringing together several duties then handled by different Government departments. It retains its funding through the Government (Marchington & Wilkinson 2003). It provides current information, independent advice and training as well as working with employers and employees to solve problems (www.acas.org.uk). The equivalent organisation in Northern Ireland is the Labour Relations Agency available at www.lra.org.uk. One of the useful services that ACAS delivers, which is related to vocational rehabilitation, is called Equality Direct. This is a confidential telephone advice service, especially designed for small businesses, providing help on managing equality issues such as disability, race, sex, age and other equality issues. This service was established in co-operation with the Equal Opportunities Commission, the Race Equality Commission and the Disability Rights Commission. The service is accessed at telephone number +44 (0) 8456 00 34 44. The most well known scheme associated with ACAS is the arbitration service, where informal complaints can be addressed if there has been no formal complaint to an employment tribunal.

However, if a formal complaint has been made to an employment tribunal, a different approach needs to take place. Employment tribunals are judicial bodies that hear claims about matters to do with employment. These include unfair dismissal, redundancy payments and discrimination. There are regional offices in England and Wales (www.employmenttribunals.gov.uk). This website is appropriate for Scotland in spite of the different legal system in this country. In Northern Ireland the office of the Industrial Tribunals and the Fair Employment Tribunal (www.employmenttribunalsni.co.uk) is responsible for processing applications for tribunals.

If your client is considering making a formal complaint against their employer, they should seek advice from suitably qualified individuals such as specialist employment tribunal solicitors, union representatives or Citizens Advice Bureaux. Unions can give advice regarding employee rights over such things as disability leave, which can be an important issue with regards to job retention and return to work. Your client should contact their union representative to obtain the correct guidance and legal support. A recently developed website called troubleatwork (www.troubleatwork.org.uk) answers commonly asked questions about difficulties encountered at work, from how to deal with an awkward boss to dealing with getting home from work safely at night.

Workplace/employer

This sector is possibly the most important piece in the puzzle of vocational rehabilitation. Without a place to work or work to carry out there cannot be any return to work. Contact with the workplace needs to be established as early as possible in the process of either return to work or job retention. Best practice for the employer suggests that there should be a return to work policy that is implemented and supported by everyone in the workplace (HSE 2004). At present there is no legislation requiring employers to assist in an employee's return to work, but the Disability Discrimination Act 1995 does mean that the employer has to make reasonable adjustments to working conditions and arrangements. Also there are responsibilities under the Health and Safety at Work Act 1974 in ensuring the health and safety of a worker on their return to work. The HSE advises that compliance with these requirements is usually made easier if there is planning ahead of an employee returning to work or starting work if it is a new worker (HSE 2004).

Within the workplace there may a range of personnel who might be involved at different stages of job retention and return to work. Table 4.9 describes some of the potential staff involved in a workplace.

Human resources staff are generally members of the Chartered Institute of Personnel and Development (CIPD) (www.cipd.co.uk), the professional body for those involved in the management and development of people. However, many human resource tasks are not undertaken by human resources departments but by managers and supervisors in business (Marchington & Wilkinson 2003). It is important to find out who has responsibility for which aspects of absence management and return to work in a business to enable a smoother process of negotiation and facilitation. It is vital to demonstrate an understanding of the organisation and management structure to show that you (as an outsider) can integrate with the business processes.

Insurance sector

Employer Liability Compulsory Insurance (ELCI) is an insurance that all employers have to buy from a wide range of insurance companies. Business Link (www.businesslink.gov.uk) explains that employers' liability insurance

'enables businesses to meet the costs of compensation and legal fees for employees who are injured or made ill at work through the fault of the employer.'

An employee who has been injured at work due to the employer's negligence can sue the employers.

By law, an employer must have ELCI and be covered for at least £5 million. Most insurers automatically provide cover of at least £10 million and the ELCI must cover all employees in the UK. An exemption was brought in 2005 for

Table 4.9 Potential staff involved in a workplace.

Member of staff	Potential role
Human resources	Developing diversity, absence monitoring, return to work and job retention policies and procedures
	Promoting diversity positively
	Engaging in awareness training about specific health conditions and disability
	Negotiating return to work planning and reasonable adjustments and monitoring return to work of employees
	Sickness absence monitoring
	Engaging professional advice from internal or external providers if necessary
	Return to work interviews
Health and safety rep	Ensuring health and safety regulations are being followed
	Risk assessment
	Advise on health and safety planning for someone's return to work or changes in practices to maintain an employee at work
Trades union rep	Promoting diversity positively
	Engaging in awareness training about specific health conditions and disability
	Negotiating return to work planning and reasonable adjustments
	Monitoring return to work of employees
	Maintaining contact with employees who are off sick
Directors	Creating the right culture to promote diversity and vocational rehabilitation for return to work and job retention
	Engaging in awareness training about specific health conditions and disability
	Sanctioning funds to pay for vocational rehabilitation and reasonable adjustments
	Sanctioning policies to enable vocational rehabilitation and reasonable adjustments
	Membership with the Employers' Forum on Disability
Management	Ensuring that procedures are undertaken to help job retention and return to work
	Helping to create the right culture to facilitate job retention and return to work
	Promoting diversity positively
	Negotiating return to work planning and reasonable adjustments and monitoring return to work of employees
	Sickness absence monitoring and maintaining contact with employees who are off sick
	Engaging in awareness training about specific health conditions and disability

Table 4.9 *continued.*

Member of staff	Potential role
Work colleagues	Promoting diversity positively
	Maintaining contact with colleagues and friends who are off sick
	Supporting colleagues who are returning to work or struggling at work
	Engaging in awareness training about specific health conditions and disability
Occupational health services	Developing diversity, absence monitoring, return to work and job retention policies and procedures
	Promoting diversity positively
	Engaging in awareness training about specific health conditions and disability
	Employment assessments for returning employees and new employees
	Advising on when to return to work
	Advising on ill-health retirement
	Negotiating return to work planning and reasonable adjustments and monitoring return to work of employees
	Sickness absence monitoring
	Engaging professional advice from internal or external providers if necessary
	Health surveillance
Employee assistance programmes	Usually a contracted-in telephone service that can provide general counselling
In-house expertise in various departments	An employer may have departments within the business that could add expertise advice to the job retention and return to work of employees. For example:
	Engineering and work-study departments can provide advice on adjustments to equipment and machinery or on the flow of work
	Rehabilitation departments can provide advice regarding functional abilities at work and reasonable adjustments and ergonomic changes

limited companies that only employed one person who also had at least 50% ownership; and for limited companies employing close family members. Some self-employed people may be considered covered under an organisation's ELCI and specialist advice should be taken to determine if this is so in the event of a claim. The ELCI was brought in under the Employers' Liability (Compulsory Insurance) Act 1969 and it is enforceable through the HSE (Business Link website 2006). Advice leaflets are available from the HSE.

When an employee makes a claim on this insurance product, a litigation case starts and some insurance companies will offer services that will help an employee of the customer (the employer) to return to work. The insurer and the claimant solicitor acting on behalf of the injured worker will handle this process together. This system works well when insurers and claimant solicitors work together using the best practice guidelines of the Rehabilitation Code 1999. The Rehabilitation Code is not compulsory but has a spirit of co-operation and rehabilitation as its focus and it was updated in 2003 (APIL website 2004). Not all ELCI providers will therefore necessarily offer rehabilitation, and the rehabilitation that may be offered and rehabilitation providers will vary widely. However, if your client is in the process of an employer's liability claim it is worth checking if they are eligible to rehabilitation which may also involve return to work initiatives (vocational rehabilitation).

Some insurance products will include comprehensive rehabilitation and appoint someone to organise the input from a range of providers – sometimes known as a case manager. Some products will involve worksite assessments, advice to employers and negotiating return to work plans and adjustments to the work and the work environment; some products will include financial assistance to start a graded return to work. A funded work trial is one way of managing this – where the employer pays the employee for the time they are at work and the insurance company picks up the cost of the remaining normal hours (usually only the net pay). This way your client can return to work without having to lose out financially. This approach needs to be handled in conjunction with sound benefits advice.

Advice about insurance companies is available through the Association of British Insurers (ABI) (www.abi.org.uk) and information about personal injury lawyers is available through the Association of Personal Injury Lawyers (APIL) (www.apil.com).

Independent and voluntary sectors

Independent providers of vocational rehabilitation may have the skills to address workplace interventions. Table 4.3 listed some of the independent providers associated with health and social interventions and how to find the practitioners. Many of those practitioners will also be able to provide workplace interventions. In addition to those already mentioned in Table 4.3 are those practitioners in the occupational health service mentioned in Table 4.8, who often work in independent practice. To these two lists might be added access auditors and consultants. Practitioners who offer advice about disability access in the workplace are now registered with the National Register of Access Consultants (NRAC) (www.nrac.org.uk). NRAC was established in 1999 as a project of the Centre for Accessible Environments. It was initially funded by central government, and the Department for Work and Pensions and the Office of the Deputy Prime Minister, the Department for Transport and the Disability Rights Commission continue to support the Register. The NRAC website (2006) is *'a resource for those seeking professional advice on how to develop inclusive environments in accordance with the Disability Discrimination Acts 1995 and 2005.'*

Those practitioners who would provide workplace interventions from the voluntary and charitable sectors will vary in their experience and expertise in helping with workplace interventions. These might be:

- Supported employment organisations
- Training organisations
- Job brokers
- Assistive technology advisors

There are a huge number of charities in the UK, too many to mention all the relevant ones in this book. Table 4.10 suggests some examples of organisations in this sector and their contact websites. Other places to obtain relevant information about this sector are your local community volunteer service and Jobcentre Plus.

Types of workplace interventions

A mind map of my own interpretation of vocational rehabilitation in the UK has already been presented in Figure 4.3. Figure 4.6 represents this final part of the mind map by suggesting in more detail the contributions of practitioners who might be associated with workplace interventions. The final category of engaging in work can be subdivided into:

- Engaging in education and training, including workplace training, formal and informal education, location of work, type of work, support methods and monitoring
- Engaging in returning to work, also including location of work, type of work, support methods and monitoring
- Engaging in job retention (remaining in work)

Associated with all three parts is the workplace plan.

Huang et al. (2006) conclude from their study on the factors affecting organisational responses to employees on sick leave that:

'Certain employee characteristics appear to influence the response of employers to work injuries.'

They explain that it has been understood for some time that employers' reactions to employees who are off sick can have an effect on disability outcomes. Studies comparing organisations have shown that those organisations with established policies and procedures for responding to employees who are injured, achieve

Table 4.10 Examples of organisations in the voluntary and charity sector that may assist with workplace interventions.

Organisation	Area of intervention	Website
Abilitynet is a charity that provides a comprehensive range of services on the use of information technology for people with all types of disabling conditions, for care and support professionals, employers and statutory bodies. This is unique in the UK, and probably in the world. Abilitynet provides assessments, advice, awareness education and consultancy on IT systems, workstations and web accessibility	ICT assistive technology	www.abilitynet.org.uk
Arthritis Care is a charity that provides awareness training to employers about working with arthritis	Training	www.arthritiscare.org.uk
DARE engages with disabled people to promote disability equality. They work in partnership with disabled people and organisations to enable them to provide services and improve employment opportunities and choice for disabled people	Training, consultancy	www.darefoundation.org
Dare provides a wide range of consulting and training services, to help employers benefit from the opportunities		
Disability Matters' mission is to help organisations profit from the potential of disabled people	Consultancy, training, vocational rehabilitation	www.disabilitymatters.com
The **Disabled Workers Co-operative** is a registered charity that helps disabled people to help themselves. Their aim is twofold – to raise the independence of disabled people (for those that want it) by enabling them to take an active role in the economy and achieve a greater sense of self-worth; and to raise awareness of the contribution that disabled people can make to society	Advice, database of skills and information	www.disabledworkers.org.uk
Diversity Works is part of **Scope** and aims to develop the leadership skills of disabled people to occupy senior management positions in British businesses	Training	www.diversityworks.scope.org.uk
Foundation for Assistive Technology (FAST) works with the Assistive Technology (AT) community to promote useful research and development for disabled and older people. The website has a useful database of a wide range of charity based providers	Research and development	www.fastuk.org

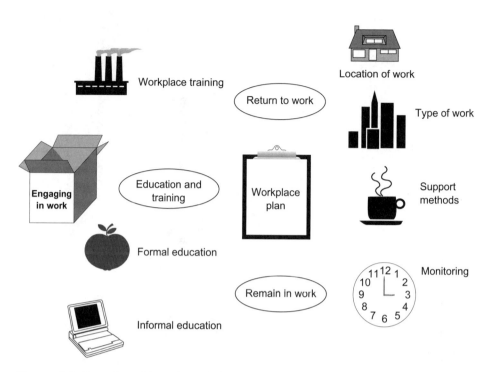

Figure 4.6 Engaging with work: workplace interventions.
Images from Microsoft Clip Art.

better outcomes in terms of employees successfully returning to work. They describe positive reactions to employees as being:

- Supportive responses from supervisors and co-workers
- Problem solving with the commitment of resources
- Job redesign and restructuring
- Efforts to enable a safe and sustained return to work

Additionally Nordqvist et al. (2003) cited in Waddell et al. (2004) suggest that good practice would include:

- The employer contacting the absent employee soon after the onset of sickness absence
- The supervisor informing the employee's co-workers about the employee off sick (without divulging confidences)
- The employer contacting the employee off sick and informing them about changes that are occurring at work
- Establishing clear routines for the return to work plan and ensuring that everyone knows who is responsible for what
- The supervisor or line manager creating a positive emotional atmosphere

Supportive responses from employers – and more importantly the supervisor or line manager – are seen as having positive effects on employees. Line managers help to interpret employer policies and keep in touch with an absent employee, giving messages that are supportive and that show concern. They have an important role in looking at adjustments to the job and to the immediate environment. However, line managers will often vary in their responses to certain employees and may not necessarily be aware of how to respond appropriately to disabled people or people with ill-health conditions. It has been shown that those employees who struggle the most with their duties at work or are dissatisfied with their job are the most likely to receive unhelpful responses from employers – and perhaps unwittingly so (Huang et al. 2006). Organisational methods that identify these people before they have an accident or take sick leave may reap rewards in helping to reduce the barriers to return to work that may be unconsciously in existence. One method already discussed in section 2 (assessments) is the Work Instability Scale by Gilworth et al. (2003).

Huang et al. (2006) reported that the most important response from an organisation was that which occurs immediately after an accident at work and it would be interesting to know if the same applies for those employees who go off sick for more than a few days. If your client went off sick from employment it is worth finding out their feelings about how the situation was handled. It may not be too late to reinstate good feelings between your client and the employer. Just making the employer aware of your client's perception of the situation may facilitate a positive response by the employer, especially if you tactfully suggest this.

Workplace plan

A workplace plan can be part of the toolkit that an employer utilises to help to create positive responses to an individual who wants to return to work or indeed start work in their organisation for the first time. Figure 4.7 shows a workplace plan situated between the three elements on the diagram of education and training, return to work and remain in work. I have put this in the middle because it is equally relevant for all three areas. If your client has needs in education and training, the workplace plan could mention how training will be integrated into returning to work; likewise, if your client has specific return to work needs or needs relevant to remaining in work, these should be mentioned in the plan. The workplace plan is, in my own view, central to ensuring adequate awareness of the needs of your client and what is required of all parties and can be especially helpful for the employer.

The workplace plan might also be called the graded return to work plan (if the return is graded), or a planned phased return to work plan or a supported employment plan. The semantics are less of an issue as long as everyone agrees the purpose of the plan. The plan might include the following considerations:

- Modifications to environment
  - Workplace equipment
  - Accessibility advice

Employer details			
Name		Line manager	
Address		HR	
		OH	
		Union	
Contact		H&S	
		Other	
Communication details: e.g. off sick contact, requires extra support contact, holiday contact:			

Employee details			
Name		Date of injury	
Address		Start of sickness absence	
Pre-absence duties			
Pre-absence job description			

Involved practitioners			
Name			
Details			
Contact			

Figure 4.7 Workplace plan/return to work plan.

Current medical certification	Date from:	Date to:
RTW plans approved by physician (name)		Date:

Goals	
RTW goals	
RTW date	

Modifications			
Area	Description	Responsibility	Required by date:
Work task			
Equipment			
Environment			
Safety considerations			

Figure 4.7 *continued.*

Training required for the employee to attend			
Employee training			
Length of training			
Onsite/offsite			
Required by date:			
Responsibility			
Contact			
Safety considerations			

Training required for individuals in the workplace to attend			
Workplace training			
Length of training			
Onsite/offsite			
Required by date:			
Responsibility			
Contact			
Safety considerations			

Figure 4.7 *continued.*

- Attitudes
- Communication channels
- Modified arrangements
  - Hours overall (finances)
  - Start and finish times
  - Location of working, e.g. home working
  - Transport to and from work
- Modified work
  - Job duties
  - Job rotation
  - Responsibilities
  - Graded return to work plan

As a demonstration of the widely varying descriptors of modified work the work of Krause et al. 1998 describes types of modified work as including the terms:

- *Light duty*. Also known as alternative duty, modified duty, restricted duty
- *Graded work exposure*. Where hours and duties are gradually increased over time
- *Work trial*. Working with an employer for a short period of time (up to six weeks or so) and where there is an arrangement for remuneration either through the employer or via Jobcentre Plus programmes
- *Supported employment*. Open employment with onsite support for the employee
- *Sheltered employment*. Paid work usually not in open employment

Figure 4.8 shows an example of a workplace plan that might also be called a return to work plan with the idea that it demonstrates the basic elements of a plan to help someone back to work. Although the plan implies that it is written for someone returning to a previous job, it can be amended to suit the organisation and the individual.

Education and training
To redress some of the imbalance with workplace issues, improving awareness and providing coping mechanisms for line managers and supervisors as well as providing interventions for an individual may be of equal importance. Shaw et al. (2003) developed a list of ideal elements to include in potential supervisor training that could enable improved facilitation of return to work. These include:

- Accommodation of temporary limitations with adjusted work
- Good communication with the employee who is off sick
- Responsiveness to queries and adjustments
- Concern over the employee's welfare
- Empathy and support offered to the employee
- Understanding and believing of the employee
- Fairness and respect provided
- Maintaining contact and follow-up

Hours of work			
	Week 1	**Week 2**	**Week 3**
Monday Date Morning Afternoon Nights Restricted duties			
Tuesday Date Morning Afternoon Nights Restricted duties			
Wednesday Date Morning Afternoon Nights Restricted duties			
Thursday Date Morning Afternoon Nights Restricted duties			
Friday Date Morning Afternoon Nights Restricted duties			

Figure 4.8   Workplace plan/return to work plan.

Saturday Date Morning Afternoon Nights Restricted duties			
Sunday Date Morning Afternoon Nights Restricted duties			
Total hours			
Prduction rates			

Monitoring			
	Week 1	**Week 2**	**Week 3**
Review date Observations Comments			
Actions Signed			

RTW Plan approval to include resources			
	Name	**Date**	**Signed**
Manager Employee Line Manager			

Figure 4.8 *continued.*

- Shared decision making
- Co-ordinating with medical providers
- Obtaining support from co-workers

Shaw et al. (2003) state:

'Interpersonal aspects of supervision may be as important as physical work accommodation to facilitate return to work after injury.'

Training ideally needs to address issues of how to empathically facilitate an employee through changes to the workplace and work. More recently, Shaw et al. (2006) report:

'Training may improve supervisors' responses to employees' reports of pain or injury, thereby improving chances for early treatment and recovery and minimising the need for time away from work.'

Awareness training may come from within an organisation such as the occupational health service, or from outside the organisation in the form of a case manager, or an organisation such as those mentioned in Table 4.10.

Other training may be recommended to the employer by a vocational rehabilitation practitioner to:

Help the workplace to accommodate their client. Training in reasonable accommodations under the Disability Discrimination Act 1995 is fairly widely available through a range of providers already mentioned in Table 4.10 and often involves education about the Act as well as case histories and problem solving contemporary accommodations for employees. Other training can be sought on specific workplace adjustments involving ergonomic changes and equipment including assistive devices. Other workplace accommodations are in the form of personal assistance services where assistance from another person compensates for a functional limitation. Training in the USA is well established in these areas where they have established vocational rehabilitation systems.

Have awareness of disability issues and diversity. Specific training to employers about diversity is available from lots of organisations and includes looking at the benefits of having a diverse workforce that includes disabled people. The training will often look at etiquette or appropriate behaviour and semantics to use with disabled people as well as looking at other employment procedures such as recruitment, selection and job retention. A thought-provoking DVD produced by the Disability Rights Commission called *The Appointment* explores attitudes to disability and working and is a good introduction to open discussions about these issues. The DVD is available from the Disability Rights website at www.drc-gb.org.

Help key people in the workplace understand a particular disability or health condition. Training in this area is much more focused around a particular employee and may be carried out on a one-to-one basis with a relevant line manager, co-workers or human resource manager. It can be used to look at specific ways to support individuals, how to spot if someone is not coping with their workload for instance, or spotting a change in mood and behaviour that may be the start of a change in their health condition. This is done with the aim of supporting an individual – not to catch them out or to instigate punitive measures. The practitioners who are involved with a client may be able to offer this kind of training as a support to the employer in the process of job retention or return to work.

Dispel common myths. More widespread education can be used as part of health promotion to dispel common myths about certain diagnoses. Myths such as, 'you can't get better from depression, once you've got it, that's it,' or 'if you have had a heart attack you shouldn't work because it's a danger to people around you,' or 'rest will help a bad back.' There are many more myths than these, of course. These sessions can be quite informal and used to improve awareness to reduce stigma and reduce fears that people may have about a colleague's safety in the workplace.

To facilitate someone returning to work. There may be some training that he or she is required to undertake with the employer:

To become reacquainted with policies, procedures and changes in the workplace during an absence. Your client might be offered the opportunity to attend some in-service training to help to reintegrate into the workplace. This might be concerned with new policies and procedures, new targets to achieve, new computer software or information management system, new equipment or introductions to a new manager. This can be a gentle way of integrating into the workplace and a way to meet colleagues and managers.

To update skills in technical areas. Updating technical skills may mean attending a formal course or training session that is externally recognised such as a NEBOSH, NVQ or degree course. Employees may be expected to attend taught sessions off the work site and they may be part of the Modern Apprenticeship Scheme, the Learning Through Work scheme or an alternative day release scheme at a local further education college.

To have licences reinstated for machinery or vehicles. This training is likely to be through formal channels and will result in a time limited 'licence to operate' type of qualification. Examples are chainsaw operators, forklift drivers, LGV drivers, 360° crane operator, piling rig and crawler crane operator. Examples of training available can be accessed through the HSE website as part of their vehicles at work area.

To obtain on-the-job training for new duties. This type of training may be carried out at a particular work site and overseen by a manager, the health and safety office or human resources. It is to orientate the employee to the job requirements and processes and can often involve well-established systematic training processes with the employer. Buddy systems might be used to teach new on-the-job skills as a way of providing support to any employee. As the practitioner, you will need to explore these training arrangements to see how they will fit with your client's needs and learning requirements.

Your client might also benefit from other informal training around managing their health condition and working and such training can be helpful in establishing coping mechanisms. Stopping work is not always the only way of coping with symptoms or challenges at work. If advice and intervention can be brought into the workplace prior to sickness absence, the appropriate coping skills and awareness training can be established.

Return to work and remaining in work

Location of working
The location in which your client chooses to work in this case refers to working at home, at an employer's facility, at a mobile location or a combination of all three. Choices may need to be made about the feasibility of your client carrying out duties in the different locations. This will depend partly on your client's needs and the particular duties that are required by the employer. Some work will only be feasible in a particular location – quite obviously driving large goods vehicles is not compatible with home working.

Working from home may be part of being self-employed or having one's own business but homeworking may be an option with an employer for some relevant duties, usually administration-based. UNISON says:

> 'Homeworking involves working at home for either part or all of an employee's contracted working hours as opposed to working in an office or other workplace. Working from home usually involves employees who are mobile for significant periods of their working time using their home as a base. These workers are also sometimes referred to as "remote workers" "home-start" or "field-start" staff.'

UNISON explains that teleworking is conceptualised slightly differently:

> 'Teleworkers are a specific type of homeworker in that they are people who work mainly at or from home and who use both a telephone and a computer to do their job.' (UNISON website 2006)

Some employees may be able to obtain equipment from their employer to carry out some duties in the home. Commonly the equipment will be a computer or a laptop, and accessories. However, homeworking might not only encompass administrative duties. As long as the work tasks are suitable for a home environment and any necessary equipment can be accommodated, it could be a possible point to negotiate. Most employers will have to follow their own policies regarding homeworking or develop some policies to ensure health and safety has been considered. Security may also be a concern for some companies and this will need investigating.

Choosing to work at the employer's facility may be the only choice that many employees will have and negotiations and recommendations may take place about adapting parts of the work environment to suit your client's needs. There are many benefits of going to a workplace. There are other people around and it is a much-enhanced social atmosphere compared with the isolation of home working. Going to a workplace separates work from home more easily, a workplace may have convenient facilities like a canteen with subsidised food, and there should be all the correct equipment and spares that are required.

Some workplaces have created special areas that are used by employees who are returning to work. These 'rehabilitation rooms or duties' are seen as a measure to assist people back into work and can be useful for some individuals for a short period. However, it is also being seen more as creating a rehabilitation ghetto in which to place people who are having trouble with their job performance, which then puts a rather negative slant on the concept. What may be required is workplace-based vocational rehabilitation using valued job duties and being facilitated by experienced practitioners. This would bridge the gap between healthcare rehabilitation and vocational rehabilitation in the healthcare setting and a real work environment.

Some types of work require the employee to be mobile and travelling around, for example sales rep, truck driver, managing director of a company, a trainer for a training company, train driver, pilot, case manager, plumber, joiner and driving instructor. Their work either is the transport of goods and people or involves undertaking work in different locations. The choices to be made about this kind of work should to be considered in line with your client's needs. If your client is skilled and motivated to return to this kind of work then there may well be assistive devices to facilitate a return to driving, or a personal assistant who can support your client as they travel around. Lone working policies and communication policies and procedures may need to be addressed. These should cover management of safety when out working alone and also cover incidents of breakdown of vehicles and other mishaps.

Type of work

As well as helping your client to integrate into the right work setting for them, you will also be involved in helping them make decisions about the type of work and working arrangements that would be suitable. Your client may be very comfortable to enter into the open competitive employment market, but he or she may not be aware of some of the other possibilities that might also seem attractive. Voluntary work is a valuable type of work for people to engage with and can give a certain flexibility that paid employment might not be able to offer. Other types of work include:

Sheltered employment. This type of employment was traditionally carried out in workshops associated with social care. Contemporary sheltered work opportunities are businesses in the open market but supplemented by grants and donations. There is debate about whether the employees get the market rate for the work they carry out and how much the job tasks are valued. However, for some people this will be the closest experience of working that they will be offered. There is a high level long-term support to clients and for some there will be the opportunity and support to move on to less supported work environment. Jobcentre Plus now calls these projects WORKSTEP rather than sheltered employment because of a focus to be able to move on to further opportunities. Remploy Ltd is the Government-run WORKSTEP project.

Supported employment. This is a concept as well as project type and is based on the idea of supporting people into open, competitive employment using natural supports that are already in the workplace. The British Association of Supported Employment (BASE) has details of providers of this type of employment.

Social firms. Social Firms UK (www.socialfirms.co.uk) aims to create employment opportunities for disabled people through the development and support of social firms. Employees are paid at market rates whatever the individual's productivity rate. Social firms are one kind of social enterprise.

Working arrangements to consider for a return to work plan are:

- Part-time working
- Full-time working
- Temporary work
- Job sharing

Your client's family circumstances may have a great bearing on what hours are suitable for them to work, especially if there are other people for whom they have responsibility. In negotiating the hours that your client works, financial implications should be discussed with the benefits advisor and the tax office if required. Changes to working hours can have an effect on claiming benefits and paying tax and National Insurance contributions.

Support methods

Support methods could include leaflets and guides, modified work, adjustments, assistive technology, ergonomic solutions and personal assistance. Employers who approach the barriers to return to work in a constructive, problem solving manner and who can also commit funds or other resources to helping someone to work may also be important in determining the future outcome of someone's employment tenure i.e. the length of employment with one organisation (Huang et al. 2006). Resources may be conceived in terms of money, but might also be manpower, for instance, to provide some support to a co-worker who needs cognitive support or physical assistance, or through a specified supported employment arrangement.

Support for employers is available in the form of leaflets and guides and some of these can be seen in Table 4.11.

Table 4.11 Examples of leaflets and guides available for employers to assist with return to work and sickness management.

Publication	Date	Publisher	Website
HSE website has a section devoted to sickness absence and return to work	N/A	Health and Safety Executive (HSE)	www.hse.gov.uk
Tackling work-related stress: a managers' guide to improving and maintaining employee health and well-being	2001	HSE (HSG218) HSE books	www.hse.gov.uk
Solutions at work: practical guide to managing recruitment	2003	Employers Forum on Disability	www.employers-forum.co.uk
Managing sickness absence and return to work in small businesses	2004	HSE (INDG399)	www.hse.gov.uk
Revitalising health and safety: case studies	Unknown	HSE	www.hse.gov.uk
Managing sickness absence and return to work: an employers' and managers' guide	2004	HSE (HSG249) HSE books	www.hse.gov.uk
Work-related stress: a short guide	2004	HSE (INDG281rev1)	www.hse.gov.uk
Tackling stress: the management standards approach	2005	HSE	www.hse.gov.uk
Working together to prevent sickness absence becoming job loss: practical advice for safety and other trade union representatives	2005	HSE (WEB02)	www.hse.gov.uk
The health and work handbook of patient care and occupational health: a partnership guide for primary care and occupational health teams	2005	Royal College of General Practitioners and Faculty of Occupational Medicine	www.facoccmed.ac.uk
Creating a healthy workplace	2006	Faculty of Public Health	www.fph.org.uk
Disability and work: a trade union guide to the law and good practice	2006	Trades Union Congress	www.tuc.org.uk

Further support for employees is available in the form of leaflets and guides and these can be seen in Table 4.12.

Adjustments and modifying work

There are legal requirements to make reasonable adjustments if an employee is, or becomes disabled under the Disability Discrimination Act (DDA) 1995. The following are factors that the DDA takes into consideration when determining if an adjustment can be called reasonable.

- Effectiveness and practicability
- Financial and other costs
- Genuine risk to health and safety
- Difficulties that relate to physical changes to premises

(www.drc-gb.org)

Further training and information on the DDA is available through the Disability Rights Commission website at www.drc-gb.org.

Modifying the work that your client carries out either on a temporary or a permanent basis is another support and adjustment that can be instigated. Krause et al. (1998) explain that there is a benefit to the employer with modified work as it has been shown to cut in half the number of days lost per disabling injury. Their results showed that there could be substantial reductions in costs associated with sickness absence. There no hard and fast rules about modifying work and it requires a unique perspective on each client. Brooker et al. (2001) say that:

'A key concern from the worker's perspective is that modified work arrangements provide a safe workplace environment that facilitates recovery from injury rather than exacerbating it.'

Often the factors to consider for change are modified working arrangements, modified work tasks and modified work environment.

Modified arrangements are the most common form of modifications (Brooker et al. 2001) and can include altering the hours that your client works. In a graded return to work, these might start off fairly short in duration but be long enough to be useful in the completion of suitable tasks. For instance, an administrator might be able to carry out a useful amount of work in half a morning at work, say, between 9.00 and 11.00, but a farm worker would need to work a full day because of the inability to stop a job part way through the day. How often your client goes into work over a graded period is also variable. The administrator might be able to start by doing half a morning three days the first week, followed by five half mornings the following week. The farm worker may have to start on two full days for the first two weeks followed by three full days over the following two weeks. There is no strict pattern to follow when upgrading someone's work.

From a practice experience point of view I find it useful to upgrade one thing at a time. For instance, if my client is upgrading his work tasks to include heavier

Table 4.12 Examples of leaflets and guides available for individuals to assist with return to work and sickness management.

Publication	Date	Published by	Website
Work Life Balance	2003	Mental Health Foundation	www.mentalhealth.org.uk
Off work sick and worried about your job? Steps you can take to help your return to work	2004	Health and Safety Executive (INDG397)	www.hse.gov.uk
Off sick? What happens and when	2004	Sheffield Occupational Health and Advisory Service (SOHAS)	www.sohas.co.uk
The comfort zone: upper limb musculoskeletal health at work. Be aware that this was written for a New Zealand audience	unknown	Burwood Academy of Independent Living, New Zealand	www.burwood.org.nz
Flexible working	2005	Advisory, Conciliation and Arbitration Service (ACAS)-(AL07)	www.acas.co.uk
Bullying and harassment at work: guidance for employees	2005	ACAS (AL05)	www.acas.co.uk
Stress at work	2005	ACAS (AL08)	www.acas.co.uk
Stop RSI – A practical guide	2006	Stop RSI	www.stop-rsi.co.uk
Return to work (after bullying) toolkit	2007	Just Fight On! Against workplace bullying and abuse	www.jfo.org.uk

Table 4.13 Example upgrading modified work for a farm worker.

Hours of work	Week 1	Week 2	Week 3
Monday Date am pm nights Restricted duties	Drilling work Full day 7.30–4.00 No lifting over 15 kg	Drilling work Full day 7.30–4.00 No lifting over 15 kg	Drilling work Full day 7.30–4.00 No restrictions
Tuesday Date am pm nights Restricted duties	No work Continue at the gym for light programme	No work Continue at the gym for intermediate programme	Drilling work Full day 7.30–4.00 No lifting over 15 kg
Wednesday Date am pm nights Restricted duties	Drilling work Full day 7.30–4.00 No lifting over 15 kg	Drilling work Full day 7.30–4.00 No lifting over 15 kg	Drilling work Full day 7.30–4.00 No restrictions
Thursday Date am pm nights Restricted duties	No work Continue at the gym for light programme	No work Continue at the gym for intermediate programme	No work Continue at the gym for intermediate programme
Friday Date am pm nights Restricted duties	No work Continue at the gym for intermediate programme	Drilling work Full day 7.30–4.00 No lifting over 15 kg	Drilling work Full day 7.30–4.00 No restrictions
Total hours	**16 hours**	**25.5 hours**	**34 hours**

NB The restricted duties would have been established at the functional assessment of this client.

duties, then I will not usually expect him to also increase his duration at work. The reason for this is the feedback I get from clients reporting how tired they feel following an upgrade. I will on occasions upgrade both duration and duties, if the client shows high self-efficacy in the duties and the ability to cope with increased duration. Another way I can see if a client is ready to upgrade duration of hours is by getting them to attend gym classes (if appropriate) in between the work days to build up stamina and get into the habit of going out every day with a purpose in mind. So you might end up with a plan that looks a little like Table 4.13.

For some people, the start and finish times are critical for being able to function at work. There are a number of prescribed medications that render people sleepy and slow in the mornings and a number of conditions where symptoms are worse on rising than later on in the day. So one technique is to establish when your client is at their best and start the graded return to work at this time and then gradually work outwards (earlier and later). So for someone who only works mornings usually, you might start them off on a half day's worth of hours from 11.00am till 3.00pm and repeat this on the days you have chosen, say Monday and Wednesday for week 1. In week 2 the upgrade could be starting at 10.30am and finishing at 2.30pm week 3 from 10.00am till 2.00pm – and so on. If your client worked full-time hours, you might want to extend the pattern at both ends so that the grading comes with an earlier start time and a later finish time.

There may be the opportunity to do a mixture of homeworking and workplace-based duties in the graded period. If this is a new development, there may well be a need for a thorough risk assessment and new policies to be considered by the employer. Transport arrangements to and from work may need to be considered in this period of upgrading. For some people in some parts of the country the drive to and from work can be exhausting. Just the drive to work could be all that someone can tolerate and this would not be a satisfactory start because they would then not easily get home again. So to overcome this, many employers will offer to pay for taxis or organise a colleague to pick up your client and drop them back home. Also, if public transport is used, this can also be an exhausting ordeal to get through before even getting to the office. Again other forms of transport might be offered for a limited period. Access to Work will also consider assisting someone with transport into work and back home again.

One important consideration in developing a graded return to work plan is that of remuneration for the employee. It should be established with the correct departments (human resources, line manager, director) what the pay structure will be during the graded return to work period. Find out if the organisation will pay the employee full wages, basic wages, or only for the hours they turn up – and how will they accrue annual leave during this period.

There is a blurring between areas of assistive technology and ergonomics and it seems to me that assistive technology is the device that someone uses and ergonomics is the science that facilitated its development and design. Assistive technology can bridge the gap between the person's functional abilities and the job requirements. The assistive technology device should be assessed for on an individual basis and the right device matched to your client. The devices can assist people when they struggle with cognitive function such as recalling events for a day or finding the way to an office; and assist people who struggle with physical function such as climbing stairs or driving a vehicle. Inge (2006) says:

'For the disabled worker AT (assistive technology) devices may be vital to obtaining employment and improving daily work performance.'

There are considered to be broadly two domains of assistive technology devices – low-tech and high-tech. Low-tech devices tend to be cheap and easily obtained in raw material form, and do not generally require training. High-tech devices, on the other hand, tend to cost more and have more sophisticated materials and electronics, be specially manufactured and often require training to use. Examples of high-tech devices might be:

- Palm-based computers
- Satellite navigation systems
- Sit-to-stand wheelchairs
- Limb prosthesis

Examples of low-tech devices might be:

- A to-do list
- Painted lines on the floor to indicate the whereabouts of the canteen
- An upturned crate as a footrest under a desk
- Fixing non-slip tape around a spade handle to improve grip

With regards to vocational rehabilitation, the assistive devices are likely to help individuals with their work tasks and getting to and from work in transport. (de Jonge et al. 2007).

It is not possible in this text to thoroughly address the wide range of ergonomic changes that might possibly be made in a workplace. The ergonomic changes that help your client are also likely to help other employees in the same workplace. So it can be a wise investment for an employer to make that will potentially reap benefits. Commonly the desk, chair, computer and immediate environment are assessed as part of the Health and Safety (Display Screen Equipment) Regulations 1992 and the miscellaneous amendments of 2002. (HSE 2003). The changes are made to ensure that the posture of the display screen equipment (DSE) user is correct to use the equipment and that the lighting and air quality are such that it is easy to see the screen. These are ergonomic changes to the work equipment. Other such changes might be replacing a regular forklift truck seat with an adjustable one that has a pneumatic seat to cushion vibrations; or a portable backrest to go in a farmer's tractor seat to give increased support in a sitting posture. Sometimes just repositioning the equipment can make the work easier to achieve.

Other ergonomic solutions can be applied to the environment, and special types of anti-fatigue flooring or matting may be put in where individuals have to ordinarily stand on concrete floors all day. Alternative handles may be fitted to doors to make them easier to open, or lighting might be improved to prevent eyestrain. The tenet is to adapt the environment and job to the workers to prevent unnecessary negative effects. In some instances, the flow of work tasks themselves will require alterations to make them less strenuous in some way. So a packaging department may need to reconsider when they undertake certain elements of the packaging line. For instance, rather than having one person doing only one element of making up a box – a very repetitive task that might cause overuse of the small wrist joints – it might be better to have the person carry out the same task but also add in a number of extra stages to the process such as taping the box up and putting in some company literature. This may well entail a shift in everyone's job tasks and possibly repositioning of parts of the packaging line, but it could mean the difference between your client returning to work and not being re-injured, and not returning to work at all.

If you have not had training in ergonomics or display screen assessments and adjustments, then you should be delegating this work to a suitably qualified person. Many practitioners with ergonomics training have other qualifications such as physiotherapy, occupational therapy and nursing.

As well as supporting your client in terms of assistive technology and ergonomic alterations, he or she may benefit from some personal assistance services (PAS). The Rehabilitation Research and Training Center at Virginia Commonwealth University (VCU-RRTC) through focus groups says:

> 'Personal assistance services in the workplace are services provided to an employee with a disability by a personal assistant to enable the employee to perform the essential duties of a job more effectively.'

The kind of assistance in the workplace may take the form of assistance with lifting and handling items from one office to another, reading handwritten letters, having a sign language interpreter at meetings, or someone to be a guide from place to place, or a reminder of tasks. The PAS can help with personal duties and work duties (Turner et al. VCU-RRTC website 2006).

Personal duties

- Assist with grooming tasks
- Assist with getting drinks
- Assist with food
- Assist with toileting
- Travel on business
- Assist with transportation

Work duties

- Making telephone calls
- Assist with filing
- Entering data
- Opening post
- Keeping the work space organised

Personal assistance in the workplace is not a new idea and is something that is facilitated by and paid for through Access to Work for disabled people. Assistance can be related to getting to work, work travel and carrying out certain tasks at work. VCU-RRTC recommends that PAS work best when they are directed by the people who use them and people with disabilities can then use these services without having to be dependent on another provider (VCU-RRTC website 2006).

For some clients, a graded reduction of supports may be an appropriate choice if there is the likelihood of improvements in physical strength, or capacity to carry out tasks, or tolerance to work in general. For instance, someone with anxiety may need support in getting to work for a number of visits while they become acclimatised to the stimulus that produces the symptom. Once exposure to the stimulus has occurred and the anxiety is no longer the problem it was, then support is no longer required. For some people who have conditions that fluctuate, there may be a cycle of requiring some support and then not requiring it. So, equipment like a crutch, splint, voice-activated software or automatic dialler might be used at some times and then stored away and not used. Sometimes transport in the form of a taxi or a driver may be required to help the individual get to work and travel for work because driving independently is not possible. However, at other times the same person may be able to safely drive and not require the extra assistance. Therefore the supports that are in place for people in the workplace need to be flexible and responsive to your client's needs. The idea of flexibility needs to be clear and communicated from an early stage in the negotiation of work with an employer.

Monitoring

Monitoring of return to work plans need to be framed in realism rather than idealism if they are to be carried out in a busy workplace, which all workplaces seem to be. It seems relevant and respectful to give as much control over the monitoring process as is feasible to your client. Retaining control seems to be a paternalistic approach that does not sit comfortably with most practitioners these days. The aim of vocational rehabilitation should be transferring to your client and their employer the ability to manage the situation of successful and sustainable return to work. That said, reviewing the client's progress is best done regularly at pre-agreed dates and times so that it remains a priority and is not sidelined by other business issues.

Monitoring return to work may continue as a process from within the employer organisation and from a combination of departments, each with their own roles. The departments in a workplace that are involved with long-term monitoring (other than return to work) are likely to be:

- Human resources
- Occupational health services
- Health and safety department or representatives
- Union representatives
- Line managers and management

Long-term monitoring in a workplace is an important part to health and safety management but can also be part of disability management systems. These systems help with job retention and can help to identify problems early on. Occupational health services often monitor the health and well-being of employees through health surveillance, sickness absence and monitoring for occupational diseases. If an organisation does not have access to occupational health, Workplace Health Connect (www.workplacehealthconnect.co.uk) and NHS Plus (www.nhsplus.nhs.uk) offer a range of services and advice such as sickness absence management, return to work rehabilitation, ill health retirement and occupational disease.

In terms of vocational rehabilitation, monitoring the workplace plan should, in most cases, be concerned with reducing the input that happens with a client, and ensuring that all parties feel comfortable with what has to happen next. The client should feel they are the one who is the expert in how they need to be supported, not the therapist. Likewise the employer should begin to feel confident that they can support their employee in productive and satisfying work. The vocational rehabilitation practitioner should be available to help out if problems arise and extra help is asked for, but many minor readjustments to the plan will be sorted out between the employer and your client – and rightly so. Minor adjustments might involve reducing hours again if a minor illness occurs, or finding that the ergonomic solution has not worked as well as hoped, or that your client is making much better gains at work and wants to increase the hours at work much quicker than anticipated. The list is endless but the little practical details can sometimes be important.

From a vocational rehabilitation service perspective, you may have permission to monitor your client's longer term and sustained return to work to gain further information about their tenure in the workplace. But it should be made very clear from the start whether this also means that extra help is also on offer if the employee or the employer reports problems.

Summary

In this chapter the interventions associated with health and social care, with career choice and skills and with the workplace have been explored. The providers of interventions have been described and suggestions have been made as to the practitioners involved and how to contact them. Interventions have been organised in categories called preparing for work, choosing work and engaging with work. It has been suggested that health and social interventions tend to reflect the preparing for work category; that career choice and skills fits in the choosing work category; and that that workplace-related interventions fit in the engaging work category.

In the UK at the moment, the industries involved in helping people to choose work is somewhat divorced from health and social care interventions (the preparation category) a gap that has been identified by contemporary research too. In vocational rehabilitation there should not be a chasm between services, a client should be able to flow backwards and forwards between relevant services to provide support when it is needed. The 21st century offers a plethora of job types and so there should – in theory – be more opportunities for disabled people if they have the right amount of support at the right time.

While there is no legislation yet requiring workplaces to instigate return to work rehabilitation in the UK there is a move to instil this concept as best practice in a diversity rich workplace. The Health and Safety Executive monitors the safety practices of workplaces and they are committed to supporting employers in job retention and return to work rehabilitation, as are other organisations such the Disability Rights Commission and the Employers Forum on Disability. One of the key messages of this chapter is the need for frequent and effective communication between all parties concerning the facilitation of people back into work.

Chapter 5

VOCATIONAL REHABILITATION SERVICES

Introduction

The vocational rehabilitation market in the UK is burgeoning with intent, meaning that it is a hot topic with potential for exponential growth of service providers. Fantastic news – except that there is a lack of structure, commissioning guidance and inter-agency design to hold all of this growth together in some sort of semblance. At the time of writing, the Welfare Reform Bill 2006 is in existence and there is great anticipation about how services might change, be structured and how vocational rehabilitation might be expected to work in the UK in the absence of any legal pressure to provide the service. This last chapter aims to explore the different elements of a vocational rehabilitation service. The material presented here is not business advice but would be more accurately described as considerations that may be relevant to start up or develop a vocational rehabilitation service.

In investigating the considerations for developing a vocational rehabilitation service, no one particular diagnostic group is featured; neither is any diagnostic group excluded. First, the past, present and future designs of vocational rehabilitation services are briefly considered to give a context in which to consider one's development of a service. Second, the practical considerations in service development are considered and include marketing, identifying the key stakeholders, commissioning and funding is considered and then referral sources are looked at. The third part is concerned with service provision and potential premises and location of premises is considered and the staff mix that may be ideally required are explored. Finally the considerations for outcome measures are explored in the context of vocational rehabilitation and service development.

At present one has to hunt for vocational rehabilitation services and then decide whether they provide the right type of service with the right amount of input and high enough quality to meet your clients' needs. Some people are better served than others. One of the least well-served groups according to Shaw et al. (2006) might be adolescents with juvenile idiopathic arthritis (JIA). They say:

> 'the provision of vocational support for young people with JIA was reported to be uncoordinated, limited and unresponsive to individual needs.'

There is no gold standard as yet or any regulatory body that monitors these services, neither is there a legal requirement to provide the service. However, these changes may yet develop with the financial strain that sickness absence and long-term disability benefits are having on the UK. Devlin et al. (2006) suggest that:

> 'The (occupational therapy) vocational service should embrace a whole continuum, ranging from day care, sheltered work, voluntary work, work experience, government schemes, open employment and training and education.'

This, together with some clear guidance on standards of practice and practitioners seems to be a good place to aim for when considering developing vocational rehabilitation services.

Vocational rehabilitation service design

Previous designs

Rehabilitation using work or occupation as a therapeutic means has been occurring since the 18th century. Phillipe Pinel in France instigated the use of tradesmen's work in the French asylum in Bicêtre with good effect. Sir William Ellis in the 19th century was concerned about the effects that poverty and unemployment had on insanity and the effect that insanity had on poverty. He also instigated the means by which the men could either follow their own trade while in hospital or learn a new trade (Paterson in Pratt & Jacobs 1997). Occupational therapy was born in the developments of these meaningful occupations and the rehabilitation became ever more refined throughout the First and Second World Wars, largely because of the pressing needs of the huge numbers of injured soldiers.

In more recent years the development of vocational rehabilitation has appeared to slow in the UK compared with other countries such as the USA or Australia and as such there is not the same range of types of intervention commonly available. A few recent vocational rehabilitation services are outlined in Table 5.1. These have been chosen to show a variety of services only and do not constitute a recommendation for the services nor a recommendation that the services mentioned here are of higher quality or effective in their outcomes.

Contemporary designs

A few current vocational rehabilitation services are now outlined in Table 5.2. As in Table 5.1 these services have also been chosen to show a variety of services only and do not constitute a recommendation for the services nor a recommendation that the services mentioned here are of higher quality than any other service or effective in their outcomes.

Future designs

The future of vocational rehabilitation will be determined in part by service user needs, research in vocational rehabilitation and lobbying authorities and the

Table 5.1 Recent vocational rehabilitation services in the UK.

Service	Outline	Further information
Remploy, UK-wide	A sheltered employment placement provider who had the majority of the placements in the UK and funded through the Government. Helped in particular those people with complex learning and physical disabilities in supported work. Remploy has now changed its focus to support more people into open employment and has demonstrated the ability to move with evidence-based practices.	www.remploy.co.uk
PACT – placement, assessment and counselling team, UK-wide	Part of the then Employment Department (now DWP) and situated in Jobcentres. This team was born out of the old Disablement Resettlement Officer role together with employment advice and workplace assistance. From this team the service has evolved (because of policy changes) into the current one of the Disability Employment Advisor and Access to Work sections, under the umbrella of the Disability Services Team in Jobcentre Plus.	www.jobcentreplus.gov.uk
NHS occupational therapy workshops, UK-wide	This was essentially rehabilitation to become work ready. There were light and heavy workshops in virtually every hospital in the UK where people could practise work skills, coming in for whole days at a time under the supervision of technical staff and an occupational therapist.	History of Occupational Therapy is available through the College of Occupational Therapists at
	Many of these workshops started declining in the early 1990s and have now almost disappeared completely, leaving a gap in rehabilitation provision. A few continue to flourish, however, and centre around rehabilitation for upper and lower limb injuries, spinal injuries and in mental health. These services have evolved and altered their practice to align with modern policies and patient needs.	www.cot.org.uk

Table 5.1 *continued.*

Service	Outline	Further information
Job retention and rehabilitation pilot (JRRP), UK selected sites	Funded through the DWP and supported by the DH, this randomised controlled trial aimed to test three different styles of intervention for people off sick from work between 6 and 26 weeks: 1) workplace-only interventions, 2) healthcare-only interventions and 3) a combination of the previous two. The project ran from 2003 until 2005 through six providers each with a different organisational structure. There were joint initiatives involving the voluntary, NHS, education and employment sectors and lots of interagency working. The teams were interdisciplinary and consisted of a wide range of professions. The project has been evaluated at a national level and the local consequences of the projects have been very positive with further vocational rehabilitation services evolving in the six areas.	www.dwp.gov.uk
Pathways to Work pilot, UK selected sites	This started in 2003 by the DWP and has essentially evolved from that point. New initiatives were introduced in seven pilot areas and included new specialist teams that involved inter-agency working. The pilot was addressing return to work for those people newly claiming Incapacity Benefit. There were new initiatives such as the return to work credit and an advisor discretionary fund as well as continuing to tap into older services such as the NDDP (New Deal for Disabled People) Job Brokers. The unique element was the introduction of the Condition Management Programme, a voluntary intervention based on symptom management and managing work.	www.dwp.gov.uk

Table 5.2 Contemporary vocational rehabilitation services in the UK.

Service	Outline	Website
Employment Opportunities, UK-wide	A charity that has been operating since the early 1980s delivering job searching and job development services to disabled people and employers across the UK.	www.opportunities.org.uk
SOHAS – Sheffield Occupational Health and Advisory Service, South Yorkshire	A charity providing, among other services, health and workplace advice and job retention and return to work case management. SOHAS also manages the Work and Health Information Gateway (WHIG) a portal with lots of information related to health and work.	www.sohas.co.uk www.whig.org.uk
Unum Provident Open Door Centres, UK-wide	This is one of a number of vocational rehabilitation services that this insurance company provides for its customers. This service is an on-site assessment and guidance centre that offers assessments of functional capacity and psychological assessments as part of determining ways to assist people to return to work.	www.unumprovident.co.uk
Skill Solutions, Jersey	This is an organisation made up of the Jersey Employment Trust, Jobscope and Workwise all based in the States of Jersey. It provides a centralised supported employment service for Jersey businesses and offers training and employment opportunities for disabled people. It provides services of assessment, sheltered employment and open employment.	www.gov.je
Papworth Trust, Cambridgeshire	This is a charity that provides a vocational rehabilitation service with a very long history, having its roots as far back as 1917. It provides a full range of interventions from assessments through rehabilitation and open employment. They have a residential and outreach services in a modular styled programme. Vocational rehabilitation is just one of a number of services it offers	www.papworth.org.uk/
TATE (through assistive technology to employment) project, Bristol	This project is about assistive technology and it is apartnership of many different organisations from different sectors. The project is looking at developing software and assistive devices that can be helpful in employment for people with learning disabilities.	www.tateproject.org.uk

Table 5.2 *continued.*

Service	Outline	Website
Breakthrough-UK, Manchester	This organisation is a charity based in Manchester and covering the north west, providing help for disabled people with job searching and career development, support, training for employers and disabled people and consultancy.	www.breakthrough-uk.com
Rehabilitation and retention service, St Helens, Merseyside	This vocational rehabilitation service is situated within an occupational health department in the NHS and only one of a few in the UK. This is a multidisciplinary team providing services to the hospital staff. It provides a comprehensive service from assessment through to rehabilitation and reintegration into work. (Langford, 2005)	www.sthkhealth.nhs.uk
VIBE, Camden, London	An early intervention, individual placement support, client-centred practice occupational therapy service based on the solution-focused approach. It is based in Camden, London for clients living in this area and the service is provided for those clients in their first episode of psychosis. This early intervention service is funded through the Camden Neighbourhood Renewal Fund. In November 2005, VIBE won the Guardian Public Service Award for the mental health category.	www.cimhscaretrust.nhs.uk
User employment services, UK-wide	This service is concerned with providing service users paid employment within the NHS Trust. Sheffield Care Trust and SW London and St George's Mental Health Trust to name two of a growing number of these initiatives in mental health. Rinaldi et al. (2004) have written about their experiences in developing a new service related to vocational rehabilitation.	NHS Trust websites
The Enable Employment Retention Scheme, Shropshire	A countywide service in Shropshire working with people with mental health problems, who may be at risk of losing their jobs while off sick from their work. Shropshire Primary Care Trust covering 48 GP surgeries and more than 200 doctors fund the service (Robdale 2005).	www.enable-shropshire.org.uk

Government to obtain the right kind of services with suitable accessibility at the right time. In part, the future of vocational rehabilitation will inevitably be determined by government policy to balance the finances of the country but will also be driven by a political ambition to improve the welfare of the country. A change in government often leads to changes in policy and eventually service design and delivery. Vocational rehabilitation is an ever-changing creature not yet governed by one authority and this is a positive attribute in the UK. This country is not yet stagnated in a bureaucratic organisation controlling the entire vocational rehabilitation market, which means there is flexibility and that change can occur swiftly to embrace new evidence-based practices or policy changes as they emerge. One thing does seem clear about the future and that is the need for service user input in all vocational rehabilitation services, current ones and those yet to develop and the need for multiprofessional and multiagency working.

The new Welfare Reform Bill 2006 has increased the scope of Pathways to Work and encourages multiprofessional and multiagency working and this seems to be embraced, as it allows smaller providers the chance to be involved as well as the larger dominant service providers. All service providers need to be aware of the whole continuum of vocational rehabilitation and not just the component that they supply. Vocational rehabilitation is not just about finding a job, or training or improving physical stamina. It is concerned with many interventions and assistance striving to help people to engage with meaningful occupations, and for some that means becoming economically active. Kirsh (2006) says:

'The larger question for rehabilitation professionals has to do with who has access to vocational services and who does not.'

The future has much to do with accessibility and visibility of services. Multiagency providers will begin to blur the boundaries between professionals and interdisciplinary teams will become the norm with occupational health, traditional healthcare, rehabilitation and employment specialists working together as teams. Vocational rehabilitation will hopefully become a commonplace service within workplaces with a particular focus on job retention and sickness absence, so developing a health promotion and disability management approach. This will give service providers the chance to work together where now they often work in parallel. For instance, a provider of an employee assistance programme (EAP) will probably have very little, if anything, to do with the physiotherapist or health and safety officer. In the future it may be more appropriate to actively include this provider in a workplace plan for an employee returning to work along with the input from the physiotherapist and the health and safety officer. This will inevitably mean closer working arrangements between the voluntary and charity sectors and the statutory and private sectors.

There are developments with regards to standards of practice and practitioner competencies for vocational rehabilitation, and there has been talk of developing a vocational rehabilitation institute for a few years now.

'The blurring of boundaries between health systems and labour policies requires a new integrating framework.' (Kirsh 2006)

Hopefully, this framework for vocational rehabilitation will not be long in coming, spurred on by organisations like the Vocational Rehabilitation Association, the National Employment and Health Innovations Network and other professional organisations. For our clients' sake it would be good to know that when we refer someone on to a particular organisation, that organisation's service delivery meets particular vocational rehabilitation standards and the staff they employ are competent to deliver the service. At present we cannot be sure that any service delivers what is says it does because there is no real transparent way of auditing them. I have had the experience myself of being very unsure whether the vocational service my client is seeing is really delivering what it says it does on the website and other than recommending to my client to cease going to the provider there is no other way of protecting her.

Innovations in technology may change the way that some interventions are delivered. Loughborough University have been researching job searching resources used by disabled people with the aim of providing an online resource to make job searching easier (*Therapy Weekly* 2006). Dannenbaum and Shaffer (2005) describe a method of using teleconferencing to help people with mental health problems in a virtual group setting. The benefits of group work for therapeutic interventions is well known and used prolifically in the NHS but not everyone can travel to a group in a particular geographical location, so developing a group using high-tech teleconferencing might be another way of reaching some people.

Perhaps one day there will be free vocational rehabilitation for everyone at the point of delivery, that provides high quality interventions through interdisciplinary teams via multiple agencies in a way that protects our (sometimes vulnerable) clients – time will tell.

Service development

Marketing vocational rehabilitation

Although many healthcare practitioners may not appreciate that their services are products and marketable, other practitioners in the vocational rehabilitation field will be aware and actively marketing their services. Marketing is not synonymous with advertising. The concept of marketing vocational rehabilitation services is no different from marketing other types of products and the process does not stop after the launch party. It is continuous to maintain planning for the future provision of the service and a marketing strategy is required for the coming years. Marketing is concerned with identifying and analysing a need and then meeting that need with a particular service or product in a way that is useful to the consumer (the person paying for the service) Table 5.3 demonstrates how this might relate to vocational rehabilitation services.

Table 5.3 A marketing process for vocational rehabilitation services.

Marketing activity	How this relates to VR
Identifying and analysing a need	Desire by employers, Jobcentre Plus and others for assistance in helping people remain in or return to work
Designing a service and product to meet that need	Specific vocational rehabilitation services and interventions to help people return to work or remain in work
Ensuring that the newly designed service and products unite with the service user so that they engage with the service or use the product	The service design is such that it attracts service users and not just the employer or another commissioner
The service is purchased and used by the customer	Customers, i.e. the employers, Jobcentre Plus, PCT etc., purchase the new vocational rehabilitation service

For further reading see Pratt and Jacobs, 1997

There are said to be four components to a marketing approach:

- Analysing market opportunities, which includes self-audit, consumer analysis and analysis of similar services and an assessment of those policies, economic factors, demographic changes (in other words, the business environment)
- Researching and selecting target markets and market segments
- Developing marketing strategies
- Executing and evaluating the marketing plan

(Pratt & Jacobs 1997)

If you are considering developing vocational rehabilitation services, you will no doubt have to go through this procedure, possibly with additional business support if you are not familiar with the processes involved with business start-ups.

To identify and justify the need for a service development a period of self-audit and gathering evidence is often required as already mentioned. Main and Haig (2006) describe an audit process they used and how they used the results to change their vocational rehabilitation intervention in an NHS setting. Through the audit process, they identified further need for continual monitoring of their service as well as refining the data they collect for the audit. The areas that Main and Haig (2006) report as auditing are:

- Client demographics – age, sex, diagnosis
- Pre-injury employment status
- Employment status on assessment
- Types of vocational rehabilitation intervention

- Post discharge employment status
- Service user awareness of the purpose of interventions
- Actual hours spent on interventions with each service user (added after the initial results were interpreted)

This is a useful insight into gathering information about a vocational rehabilitation service and in developing services it seems reasonable to try and obtain as much relevant information on other service audits as is feasible.

An alternative way of gathering relevant information was described by Devlin et al. (2006) when they went through a process of service development of their vocational rehabilitation service in Northern Ireland, called the Job Clinic. They were commissioned by an NHS managers group to provide an overview of the vocational rehabilitation service. To gather information about the relevant services in Northern Ireland, they arranged a consultation meeting – a focus group of sorts – using-open ended questions in a questionnaire as well as gathering demographic information including:

- Number and grades of staff (this would also give you information on wages costs)
- Number of referrals in a given year
- Referral source
- Referral criteria
- How well the service adhered to their model of vocational rehabilitation service (job clinic model)

Once the information was collated, a SWOT analysis (strengths, weaknesses, opportunities, threats) was undertaken to make sense of the detail before making recommendations to develop the job clinic model across Northern Ireland. Devlin et al. (2006) say the process was lengthy but worthwhile, and had the desired effect of information gathering and developing the services further.

Additional information might be required about relevant staff qualifications, experience and expertise. The NHS Key Skills Framework, by which all jobs are measured, will be a useful starting point for these kinds of demographics.

Key stakeholders

In Chapter 4, vocational rehabilitation and the sectors in which it can sit were illustrated in Figure 4.1 and the sectors associated with provision of vocational rehabilitation services were described in Table 4.1 – these sectors are the key stakeholders. In summary they can be anyone or any organisation that has:

- Employees who could potentially have sickness absence or struggle at work
- Service users who would like to return to work or start work for the first time

The stakeholders extend from the individual service users to government departments and everyone in between. The local stakeholders' names will differ in each locality, so you should research who your local stakeholders are as well as those nationally-based ones. Table 5.4 suggests how to start finding your own named people relevant for your location.

Table 5.4 Accessing stakeholders in vocational rehabilitation.

Sector	Potential stakeholder	Website
Service user	The individual/employee	
Parliament	Your local members of parliament	
Primary care trust (PCT)	The GP in a surgery, the practice manager	
The NHS (mostly secondary care)	The local hospitals' executive committee and the managers of rehabilitation departments	
	The local strategic health authority	
Local authority (LA)	The local councillors, the chief executive of social services, disability champions	
Voluntary organisations	Council for voluntary service	www.navca.org.uk
Private vocational rehabilitation companies	Chamber of commerce, local branch of the Federation of Small Businesses, professional organisations that advertise members, RehabWindow	www.chamberonline.co.uk www.fsb.org.uk www.rehabwindow.net
Insurance providers	The Association of British Insurers, Chamber of commerce, Yellow Pages directory	www.abi.org.uk www.chamberonline.co.uk www.yell.com
Legal sector	Association of Personal Injury Lawyers, chamber of commerce, Yellow Pages directory	www.apil.org.uk www.chamberonline.co.uk www.yell.com
Employers	Chamber of commerce, yellow pages directory	
Education sector	Further education colleges, special Educational Needs Co-ordinators in Connexions, Local Education Authority Managers	www.connexions-direct.com
Department of Work and Pensions (DWP)	Jobcentre Plus offices, the Disability Services Manager, The Disability Employment Advisor, The Access to Work Advisor, The Personal Advisors for Pathways to Work initiatives, Condition Management Programme Managers	www.dwp.gov.uk www.jobcentreplus.gov.uk

Table 5.4 *continued.*

Sector	Potential stakeholder	Website
	The Jobcentre Plus may also have a list of all the organisations it contracts in the private and voluntary sector to provide interventions	
Health and Safety Executive	Local health and safety representatives in organisations, Sickness Absence and Return to Work unit	www.hse.gov.uk
Department of Health	Department leads who deal with occupational health, and liaise closely with DWP. At a local level policies and targets will be translated into hospital and PCT targets	www.dh.gov.uk
Trades unions	Local union representatives	

Commissioning and funding

Commissioning in this sense is about placing an order for a particular service or set of interventions. This will usually occur through particular people or committees who are authorised by their organisation. So in a primary care trust, a particular GP practice can now undertake commissioning, a function granted through the Department of Health. Commissioning of vocational rehabilitation services may come from some of the stakeholders already mentioned. In my view the most likely in this early part of the 21st century is Jobcentre Plus, through GPs' practice-based commissioning and insurance companies. Jobcentre Plus has targets to reduce the number of claimants on what was the Incapacity Benefit and will be the Employment and Support Allowance (from January 2008). In 2006 the Government set a target of reducing benefit claimants by one million over 10 years. One way it is hoping to accomplish this is through the new Pathways to Work programme, which is being rolled out to all areas in England, Scotland and Wales by April 2008. From October 2007, private and voluntary sector providers will help deliver the Pathways service to the remaining 60% of incapacity benefits customers (DWP website 2006).

The Department of Health produced guidelines in February 2006 for commissioners on the commissioning of vocational services for people with severe mental health problems, which was an action point within the *Mental Health and Social Exclusion* report and the *Choosing Health* White Paper. The Department of Health (2006) explains the foundation commissioning principles are:

- Priority is accorded to enabling people to retain and gain paid employment and mainstream education, including the provision of support to retain and gain employment/education.
- Where it is not possible for a person to access paid employment due to the extent of their support or supervision needs, or there is an individual preference not to access paid employment, then access to mainstream education and voluntary work is needed.

This guidance is particularly useful because it is the first of its kind and will hopefully be followed by more guidance appropriate for people who have other long-term health conditions and disabled people. The guidance is also useful because it helps service providers look at their services in a positive way to enable them to develop in line with what commissioners are looking for.

In many situations where you are setting up a new service, you may be able to tap into funding through tenders where an organisation might advertise in a sense to potential service providers about a particular service or product need. There are some organisations in the UK who concern themselves with supporting new small business ventures, voluntary sector ventures, social enterprises and charities. Two of these are:

- j4b plc (www.j4b.com) describe themselves as, 'an information services company offering research, information publishing, technology and business services to a wide range of public and private sector clients in the UK and abroad. j4b is Europe's expert provider of public funding resources, conducting research into public funding and publishing grants databases. We provide technology solutions that support both grant administrators and grant applicants.'
- Direct Support (www.directsupport.org.uk) 'is one of the longest running support services for UK online centres. We have been helping centres since 2000. A free guidance and mentoring service, DirectSupport is now funded by Ufi. Regular updates and commentaries on funding are provided within the DirectSupport online service, and Experts Online will provide funding searches and advise on strategies and sources. We also help with developing plans for funding, sustainability and business planning.'
- Supply2.gov.uk (www.supply2.gov.uk) explains that this 'is the first portal of call to consolidate access to lower-value opportunities from across the whole of the UK public sector.' This service is part of the Department for Trade and Industry.
- The new Pathways to Work programme-tendering process required the potential service providers to go through an accreditation process, which among other things required the service provider to show that they were financially robust and had evidence to show that they could deliver the programmes they were presenting (Frost & Reel 2006). Whatever funding you elicit, such as community regeneration, European or Department of Health funding, it is highly likely that you will be asked to provide hard numbers about how their money will be used in your service. For this you need to have a sound business plan

with a strong financial basis, showing where in the business the money will potentially be spent, demonstrating value for money and that your service will be able to survive and not go bankrupt. This is no different from, for example, engaging childcare services for our children – we need to know that the nursery will not go bankrupt leaving us high and dry with no care.

It has not been possible to locate any published material on how to cost out a vocational rehabilitation service, and as such parallel service costs have been explored. The UK Home Care Association (www.ukhca.co.uk) was funded to undertake a costing project for the Department of Health in 2002 and in its initial paper proposed an analysis of costs for home care that would eventually produce a costing model. The costing model (in Microsoft Excel) can be downloaded at www.ukhca.co.uk. The costing model takes a

'broad range of operating costs, salaries and other expenses and uses them to calculate a cost per hour of service provision.' (UKHCA Costs Calculator for Home Care)

UKHCA explains that the costing model leads you through a process in a user-friendly manner to input information on current work commitments:

'For example: the direct hours of care provided, the number of service users, the number of visits, the timing of visits (time bands), travel (distance and time).'

The costing model then asks for additional information to be added regarding staff resources

'including the posts in the organisation, their roles and the hours they work, the time spent on management and/or client care, non-contact time.'

The costing model then factors in on-costs such as

'induction and basic training, ongoing training and supervision, leave and sickness costs, unsocial hours, etc.'

Finally, indirect costs, such as office accommodation, equipment, marketing, etc. are added into the equation. The breakdown of costs for the home care service or proposed home care service enables open discussion between providers and commissioners

'as a means of negotiating the price of providing services by using justifiable cost components.' (www.ukhca.co.uk)

Although this model is for the home care market, it is comparable in service make-up and it is provided here as a very useful indicator of how to explore costs associated with a service industry. Much of the vocational rehabilitation work is comprised of visiting service users at home or at work. The additional factors to consider are seeing service users in groups and costs associated with this, compared with individual work and potentially larger premises with a clinic-type area to house rehabilitation equipment.

The purpose of raising awareness of this particular model is to demonstrate a user-friendly tool for practitioners who might otherwise be unaware of all the potential costs associated with developing a service.

Potential commissioners of vocational rehabilitation are:

- Department for Work and Pensions
- National Health Service
- Primary care trusts
- Insurance companies
- Solicitors
- Small to medium enterprises and other employers locally and nationally
- Health and Safety Executive

If you are considering developing your vocational rehabilitation service, then looking wider than your own organisation for funds may reap benefits in obtaining multiagency funding to deliver services. This is particularly true if you currently sit in an organisation that is losing money. Your potential development needs to sit easily within the boundaries of these other organisations' policies and key targets they have to meet.

In vocational rehabilitation in the UK you need to be fully aware of the Welfare Reform Bill and all the changes that are occurring as a result of that. For instance the Cities Strategy is one element of Welfare Reform. It aims to tackle worklessness in the most disadvantaged communities across the UK. The strategy is based on the idea that local partners (a consortium) can deliver more if they combine and align their efforts behind shared priorities, and are given more freedom to try out new ideas and to tailor services in response to local need (DWP website 2006). More information about the Welfare Reforms can be obtained through the DWP website (www.dwp.gov.uk/welfarereform).You should be aware of all policy changes in government to be one step ahead of your competitors, so keep abreast of what is happening especially in the:

- Department for Work and Pensions (DWP)
- Health and Safety Executive (HSE)
- Department of Health (DH)
- Department of Trade and Industry (DTI)
- Department for Education and Skills (DfES)

Research your potential commissioner and find out all about them, what their targets are, how to speak their language and how you can sell your idea in a way that makes them see you are there to help them deliver their aims. It is not rocket science but it does involve lots of planning and research, if you want to obtain the right funding.

Referrals

You may already have an idea of where you would like your referrals to come from and you may be in a financial position to pick and choose whom you accept referrals from. However, if your funding comes from a particular source such as a GP practice, they may dictate the source of the referral as well as the criteria for the referral. So in one vocational rehabilitation business with several sources of funding, you may develop variable streams through which certain types of people flow. The more complicated it is, the more administration time will need to be spent on ensuring that you do actually obtain the payment for seeing your clients.

Ideally, of course we would like to be able to develop a vocational rehabilitation service that anyone off the street with a particular return to work need could come in to and obtain the services at no cost to them at the point of delivery. However, this is highly unlikely to occur and so how you accept your referral needs refining, based on:

- Your funding
- The clients or service users you hope to attract
- The services you supply
- Your staff mix and expertise
- Your resources in terms of space and equipment
- The time you have to offer your service users

So referrals could come from (in no particular order) the service user, Jobcentre Plus, an employer, human resources, the service user's family, health and safety officer, GP, occupational health services, solicitors, insurers, other vocational rehabilitation services, voluntary and charity sector organisations, private healthcare companies, the NHS, a primary care trust or consortia of businesses interested in helping people back to work.

Service provision

Premises

Choosing the right kind of premises is important, so that your developing service will be able to grow and not be stifled in five years' time. The kind of premises you choose will depend on what you want to use them for. If your particular vocational rehabilitation service is going to provide one-to-one talking therapies, then your requirements will be totally different from providing functional capacity evaluations (FCE) and work simulation. Your service may be looking for large industrial units or small private and soundproof offices. You will need to consider where your staff and your clients will park if they drive to your facility and free parking spaces may be seen as an added bonus to the service user.

The type of premises requirements suggested here are for those facilities that want to have the space to provide a broad range of vocational rehabilitation including FCEs, work hardening, and conditioning as well as space for one-to-one interventions. What is described here is not necessarily what your service will end up with and is just a guide of what to consider.

Approximately 1500–3000 square feet (140–279 square metres) to accommodate 6–12 clients carrying out work hardening and work simulation activities on a 4–8 hour basis per day based on advice from Matheson Associates (2002). A unit that has a loading dock is useful for simulating this type of work and stairs are useful to accommodate further cardiovascular work and mobility training. A split-level unit with offices on the upper level and one entire space underneath is also a useful option. A minimum height for the space would be 12 feet (3.5 m). Rental of spaces this large in industrial areas commands rents well in excess of £8000 per annum (March 2007). Ideally, there should be accessibility to use the space outside the unit to simulate certain activities outdoors, for instance shovelling or digging. Likewise there should be as much natural light within the unit as is possible. Most industrial units do not have many windows, so this may not always be possible. If natural light is not possible, then lighting and bulb types need to be considered carefully and ergonomic advice may be worthwhile obtaining. There should be separation of dirty and clean spaces and likewise separation of quiet and noisy spaces.

Your vocational rehabilitation service may benefit from a waiting and reception area, staff offices, staff room, showers, industrial sink areas, toilets, storage areas, quiet rooms in addition to the space required for the active rehabilitation work. Think about the type of flooring – ideally it would be sensible to have a range of floor types like concrete, linoleum, carpet together with some specialised flooring or mats such as the anti-fatigue mats for standing work.

For the specific assessments and rehabilitation the facility will have to have a range of appropriate pieces of equipment such as mentioned in Chapter 2. Many of these assessments can double up as rehabilitation equipment, and while some of the rehabilitation equipment is readily available in the UK, other pieces such as specialised work hardening equipment may need to be imported from the USA. To have an idea of the range of rehabilitation including vocational rehabilitation equipment available visit the website for AliMed at: www.alimed.com. The equipment you have in your facility may require personal protective equipment to improve safety and so a supply of overalls, steel toe-capped boots, eye protection, ear protection, hard hats, gloves and gauntlets, knee protection, high-visibility vests and waterproof outerwear may be required. A wide range of safety equipment is available through the Internet and local outfitters that deal with work wear.

The arrangement of activities and equipment is based on the risk of injury and the riskier the activity the closer it should be to the main office areas. There should be an open plan area for an office within the work hardening area. Clinical interventions such as acupuncture and injections require special guidance to be followed regarding the type of suitable environment and the disposal of sharps.

There are many safety considerations when developing a facility that includes work hardening and professional advice from an architect, surveyor and health and safety consultant is essential, as is the need to obtain advice from your local planning department on whether you will be allowed to use the building for your intended purpose. Your facility will have to meet the Disability Discrimination Act requirements on accessibility – the Centre for Accessible Environments (www.cae.org.uk) can provide advice and training on this topic.

Your facility will need to abide by all the HSE regulations and guidance on health and safety at work and you will need to spend time carrying out risk assessments for all the equipment and many of the activities in the building.

What are not mentioned here are the computing and electrical and plumbing requirements of the facility – this will depend more on which interventions you are expecting to deliver, but should not be forgotten. For instance, if you need to have a cooker, fridge, sink, or dishwasher in your facility to simulate kitchen work, this should be considered at the outset and not after all the plans and designs have been drawn up.

Location

The location of your facility will be somewhat dictated by your budget, the local area in which the vocational rehabilitation service is to be established and the local transport links. Ideally the facility should be located near to public transport with a footpath to the facility at least. You may decide that your facility would be best placed near other related services like the leisure centre or a Jobcentre Plus office, or a hospital. If you have a choice of location, take time to consider this and canvass local stakeholders for their opinions as they might be more willing to make referrals and supply funding if you are on their doorstep. The vocational rehabilitation does not necessarily need to be in one location and could be spread across a geographical area, making use of the diversity that a local population and locality gives. Your vocational rehabilitation service may comprise consultants based all over the country delivering the interventions on site into people's workplaces and homes.

For some elements of vocational rehabilitation, an industrial setting will be appropriate, for some a business complex will be right, for others a leisure complex or medical centre or community centre may be what is called for. Perhaps your facility could be a mobile one, travelling to different rural areas to provide interventions. There is no one place which is best and it depends what you are planning to deliver.

Staff mix

The success of getting back to work or retaining your client in their job depends on co-operation between all the players involved in vocational rehabilitation. Waddell et al. (2004) advise that everyone involved must *'share a common approach to management, which depends on common understanding, perceptions and attitudes to common health problems and their relation to work.'*

This means that communication between all parties is vital. Waddell and Burton (2004) also suggest that it is communication that has the greatest scope for improvement and that the greatest scope for improvement and that the greatest obstacle to this is

'the lack of knowledge and understanding of occupational issues by doctors and therapists, and of common health problems by employers: the greatest need is for each to develop an interest in the other's perspective.'

Pransky et al. (2004) take this one step further:

'Improvements in communication may be responsible for success across a variety of new interventions. Communication-based interventions may further improve disability outcomes.'

It is debatable who should make up a suitable team for vocational rehabilitation intervention. It is highly unlikely that any one service will have the exact mix correct but determining what the right mix of staff is appropriate for your service is important. Staff from different professional backgrounds and with different areas of expertise will probably have different understanding of the issues related to vocational rehabilitation. This is good in most ways because there is a broad range of people to deal with the broad range of issues that clients will bring to the service elements of a vocational rehabilitation service.

Pransky et al. (2004) advocate a situation where communication is multidirectional, not authoritative and where it is continual and effective. All players include the client (service user) and the employer in the make-up of the team. This also means that there will need to be a period of time spent on team building and building awareness and an appreciation of each other's expertise.

The potential staff may come from the following types of backgrounds:

- Service user
- Health
- Social care
- Rehabilitation
- Health and safety
- Technical
- Business/employer
- Welfare rights and finance
- Education
- Research
- Administration

The vocational rehabilitation interventions and service that you provide will demand a certain mix of people with these backgrounds. Using a framework like the NHS Key Skills Framework to determine which skills and knowledge your service needs and what kind of person you require will translate into recruiting and selecting the right people. An alternative method of exploring skills and knowledge has been supported by Hagner et al. (2002). They report that a system of using critical incidents was used to develop a list of competencies for staff working in vocational rehabilitation. This method, they said, reflected the subtle skills and knowledge that other methods had not previously identified in regards to staff working in job development and employment specialist roles (comparable to those roles in job brokerages in the UK). It is highly unlikely that one kind of profession will be able to provide all elements for the service. The suggestion from Main and Haig (2006) from their experience was to look at developing a skill mix, where a supervisor can take the lead and oversee other staff of lower grades or those with less experience.

The number of staff a service takes on is often a financial decision based on what can be afforded, because the major costs for any service are those related to salaries and on-costs. More numbers of the same kind of staff may increase capacity to see clients and the same number of staff with a skill mix may mean that the service can offer a wider range of services, but not necessarily any more efficiency.

As a sole trader, I can manage comfortably a caseload of 15–20 clients. However, I am also responsible for all of my own administration, financial responsibilities and service development. If I also employed an administrator I might be able to increase that caseload, but I would not necessarily be able to provide any wider interventions than I already do. If I joined forces with another occupational therapist with different skills, then together we could increase the services we provided but I would not necessarily be able to increase the numbers of clients on my caseload. Current service providers vary in size and in what services they offer in the vocational rehabilitation continuum. If one service were to offer all the elements of vocational rehabilitation in one facility, it would be a sizeable organisation in its own right.

Outcome measurement

Measuring the success of a vocational rehabilitation service is of the utmost importance these days and outcome measurement is the measure that is used.

'Outcomes function by providing a framework for understanding the person, addressing the full range of issues that may be important to people is essential to ensuring that work supports compliment other activities in the person's life.' (Gardner & Campanella, in Pratt & Jacobs 1997)

To understand the person, the vocational rehabilitation service needs to involve that person in describing what the important issues are – and then to provide interventions and supports to achieve their goals. So the service is person-centred. In support of this sentiment from Gardner and Campanella, Butterworth (2005) has developed, together with colleagues around the UK

'the guiding principles and practice, which govern good job retention services.'

There are 10 guiding principles written specifically for mental health services and these are:

- Early intervention dramatically improves the possibility of people returning to work.
- Case managers are effective in assuming some burden of responsibility during the process.
- Assessments are essential in providing a complete picture of the client's life at the time of referral.
- A collaborative individual planning process provides a vital foundation for effective service delivery.
- Mental health is all about relationships and supporting the naturally occurring support.
- The case manager ensures that all agencies 'sing from the same hymn sheet'. They are assessors, negotiators, mediators and problem solvers but they are also keenly aware of their limitations.
- Case managers have a professional background in mental health. Whether they work for a healthcare trust, a voluntary organisation or in the private sector, they need close ties with mental health services.
- Case managers must be familiar with the Disability Discrimination Act and health and safety legislation.
- Job retention services present opportunities for meaningful mental health education.
- Sometimes it is better to help someone find a new career path, rather than return to the old job.

Although these are written for mental health service providers, they are useful guiding principles for all job retention services and person-centred practice. Gardner and Campanella in Pratt and Jacobs (1997) go further to say when service providers look

'beyond work tasks to the direct and indirect outcomes that people expect from work, success and quality in employment services is defined by responsiveness to individual need.'

So outcome measures need to allow flexibility in a service to provide individual programmes of support and rehabilitation. An overly processed service often results in pigeonholing people into particular programmes and streams of rehabilitation and do not respond to the uniqueness of each service user.

Including service users in the development of services is a grounded approach to exploring the right mix of outcome measures for the service. This was an approach that was used by the Council on Quality and Leadership in Supports for People with Disabilities (formerly known as the Accreditation Council) in the USA in the early 1990s, when they developed their outcome-based performance measures (Accreditation Council 1993 cited in Pratt & Jacobs 1997). This outcome measure is used in services that are accredited with the council, including some organisations in Ireland and Australia as well as those within the USA.

Traditionally, outcomes for vocational rehabilitation looked at employment outcomes and for the organisations that fund these services, this remains important data to collect. Traditionally the outcome measure has been:

- Return to same job, same employer
- Return to same job modified, same employer
- Return to different job, same employer
- Return to same job, different employer
- Return to same job modified, different employer
- Return to different job, different employer
- On the job training
- New skill training or retraining
- Other educational/academic program

(New Hampshire Department of Labor, USA website 2006)

This kind of outcome doesn't tell you about the personal gains that an individual has made, if any, while engaging with your service. Organisational outcomes measures tend to be more rigid and reflect processes within a vocational rehabilitation service. Quality measurement is usually based on input–process–outcome (Gardner and Campanella in Pratt and Jacobs 1997). Inputs are those resources that a service has allocated to it to support the service user, such as:

- Facility, building and equipment
- Number of staff, qualifications, experience
- Budget allocated
- Assessment tools and resources
- Staff knowledge base

The organisational processes are how the resources are used, for instance:

- The service is provided in the way it reports it should have been provided.
- The service provides its service in compliance with relevant laws, regulations, guidance and contract stipulations. Contracts may stipulate that contact with a service user is carried out within 36 hours, assessment appointments must be arranged within 24 hours of receiving a referral, the goals must be arranged with the service user and signed or that records must be kept in a lockable cabinet.

- The organisational outcome measures are those outcomes produced by the vocational rehabilitation service. If the vocational rehabilitation service is accredited with a particular organisation, it will set their own standards in terms of outcomes. This is where the outcomes can end up being a set of data about the demographics, rather than the individual quality of the outcome. The outcomes should be related to the services that have been provided. For example, if a vocational rehabilitation does not address cardiovascular fitness for work, then it cannot measure an outcome for this. Outcomes might be in terms of improved functioning in the psychological, physical and social dimensions of a person's life, but these then need to be addressed as an input to the programme.

Taking the traditional hierarchy above, it cannot be determined if the service users who returned to same job–different employer felt that this was a good outcome for them. Likewise, if through accreditation the service needs to collect data about how many service users were seen for assessment within the time parameters, this does not demonstrate the quality of the assessment. What is needed is a blend of the two approaches, outcomes that look both at the 'how many?' elements and the 'did it meet the services users' needs?' elements.

The Department of Health (2006) produced guidelines for commissioners of vocational services for people with severe mental health problems – within these is a section on monitoring and effectiveness. The guidance suggests a blend of the statistical information as well as the quality outcomes from the service user. The guidance explains that:

> 'Involving people with severe mental health problems in the monitoring of vocational services can offer a helpful perspective on the effectiveness of those services. People themselves are the best judges of whether current services are meeting their vocational needs, preferences and choices.'

For many current services in the UK another user of the vocational service is the employer and it is therefore very relevant to include employers in the discussions about the development of outcome measures. The Department of Health guidance goes on to suggest that outcomes provide a measurement of the effectiveness of vocational rehabilitation services, and that outcomes can be measured against the number or proportion of people:

- Gaining paid employment
- Retaining paid employment
- Using permitted work
- Supported to gain/retain employment in public services (e.g. mental health trusts, PCTs, local authorities)
- Supported in mainstream education
- Supported in integrated voluntary work
- Small business enterprises

In vocational rehabilitation it is important to remember that the services are provided to support people in obtaining their own personal outcomes:

> 'People work to achieve individual outcomes. Work is not an end in itself.'
> (Gardner & Campanella in Pratt & Jacobs 1997)

The outcome measures need to reflect the individuality of the experience of the service user and provide evidence that the service is achieving the claims that are made in advertising material.

Summary

In Chapter 5 the various elements of a vocational rehabilitation service have been explored a little. In investigating the considerations for developing a vocational rehabilitation service the past, present and future designs of vocational rehabilitation services have been briefly considered to give an idea of the range of services. The practical considerations in service development include marketing, identifying the key stakeholders, commissioning and funding and then referral sources. The next part looked at service provision and potential premises and location of premises has been considered as well as the staff mix that may be required. Finally, the considerations for outcome measures have been considered in the context of vocational rehabilitation and developing a service.

Vocational rehabilitation, like other rehabilitation, is and will continue to be a developing field of practice with inevitable changes in interventions based on new evidence that is gained through research and also through outcome measurements. It is vital, therefore, that services are thought out carefully and systematically to provide the right kind of service for each individual who uses the service, whether they are an employer or a potential employee, and to ensure that the vocational rehabilitation service is an exemplar in a healthy workplace. The detail in this section cannot be construed as business or legal advice and is here to provoke thought and consideration to the variables involved in developing a vocational rehabilitation service, however large or how small it is.

WEBSITE ADDRESSES

Here is a list of the organisations mentioned in this book, and their acronyms. All the websites were accessed between February 16–19, 2007.

Website address	Organisation	Abbreviation
www.abilitynet.org.uk	Abilitynet	
www.acas.org.uk	Advisory, Conciliation and Arbitration Service	ACAS
www.agencycentral.co.uk	Agency Central	
www.alimed.com	AliMed	
www.amicustheunion.org	AMICUS	
www.arthritiscare.org.uk	Arthritis Care	
www.abi.org.uk	Association of British Insurers	ABI
www.acpohe.org.uk	Association of Chartered Physiotherapists in Occupational Health and Ergonomics	ACPOHE
www.adp.org.uk	Association of Disabled Professionals	ADP
www.anhops.com	Association of National Health Occupational Physicians	ANHOPS
www.aohnp.co.uk	Association of Occupational Health Nurse Practitioners	AOHNP
www.apil.com	Association of Personal Injury Lawyers	APIL
www.barrierfree-recruitment.com	Barrierfree-recruitment.com	
www.breakthrough-uk.com	Breakthrough UK	
www.babcp.com	British Association for Behavioural and Cognitive Psychotherapies	BABCP
www.afse.org.uk/	British Association for Supported Employment	BASE
www.babicm.org	British Association of Brain Injury Case Managers	BABICM
www.basw.co.uk	British Association of Social Workers	BASW
www.chamberonline.co.uk	British Chambers of Commerce	BCC
www.bps.org.uk	British Psychological Society	BPS

www.burwood.org.nz	Burwood Academy of Independent Living, New Zealand	
www.businesseye.org.uk	Business Eye (Wales)	
www.bgateway.com	Business Gateway (Scotland)	
www.businesslink.gov.uk	Business Link	
www.cimhscaretrust.nhs.uk	Camden and Islington Mental Health and Social Care Trust	
www.caot.ca	Canadian Occupational Performance Measure (Canadian Association of Occupational Therapists)	COPM
www.caninepartners.co.uk	Canine Partners	
www.csip.org.uk	Care Services Improvement Partnership	CSIP
www.crac.org.uk	Careers Research and Advisory Centre	CRAC
www.careers-scotland.org.uk	Careers Scotland	
www.careersserviceni.com	Careers Service Northern Ireland	
www.careerswales.com	Careers Wales	
www.cmsuk.org	Case Management Society	CMSUK
www.cae.org.uk	Centre for Accessible Environments	CAE
www.usq.edu.au/users/machin/cwb.htm	Changing Wonky Beliefs	
www.charity-commission.gov.uk	Charity Commission	
www.cipd.co.uk	Chartered Institute of Personnel and Development	CIPD
www.cochrane.org	Cochrane Library	
www.cot.org.uk	College of Occupational Therapists	COT
www.otip.co.uk	College of Occupational Therapists Specialist Section: Independent Practice	OTIP
www.communitiesscotland.gov.uk	Communities Scotland	
www.cbi.org.uk	Confederation of British Industry	CBI
www.connexions-direct.com	Connexions	
www.darefoundation.org	DARE Foundation	DARE
www.dash.iwh.on.ca	DASH Outcome Measure (Institute for Work and Health, Canada)	DASH
www.dfes.gov.uk	Department for Education and Skills	DfES
www.delni.gov.uk	Department for Employment and Learning, Northern Ireland	DELNI
www.dsdni.gov.uk	Department for Social Development, Northern Ireland	DSDNI
www.dft.gov.uk	Department for Transport	DfT
www.dwp.gov.uk	Department for Work and Pensions	DWP

www.dh.gov.uk	Department of Health	DoH
www.dialuk.info	Dial UK	
www.directsupport.org.uk	Direct Support	
www.disabilityalliance.org	Disability Alliance	DA
www.diss.org.uk	Disability Information Service	DISS
www.disabilitymatters.com	Disability Matters	
www.dptac.gov.uk	Disabled Persons Transport Advisory Committee	DPTAC
www.disabledworkers.org.uk	Disabled Workers Co-operative	
www.disabledgo.info	DisabledGo.info	
www.diversityworks.scope.org.uk	Diversity Works	
www.do-it.org.uk	Do-It	
www.drfoster.co.uk	Dr Foster	
www.employers-forum.co.uk	Employers' Forum on Disability	EFD
www.ento.co.uk/	Employment National Training Organisation	ENTO
www.opportunities.org.uk	Employment Opportunities	
www.enable-shropshire.org.uk	Enable Shropshire	
www.epicrehab.com	EpicRehab (USA)	
www.ergonomics.org.uk	Ergonomics Society	
www.epr.be	European Platform for Rehabilitation	EPR
www.expertpatients.nhs.uk	Expert Patients	
www.facoccmed.ac.uk	Faculty of Occupational Medicine	FOM
www.fph.org.uk	Faculty of Public Health	FPH
www.fsb.org.uk	Federation of Small Businesses	FSB
www.fastuk.org	Foundation for Assistive Technology	FAST
www.n-i.nhs.uk	Health and Care NI	
www.hse.gov.uk	Health and Safety Executive	HSE
www.health-and-work.gov.uk	Health and Work (uk government website)	
www.wales.nhs.uk	Health of Wales	
www.healthscotland.org.uk/hwl	Healthy Working Lives (Scotland)	
www.hie.co.uk	Highlands and Islands Enterprise	
www.hmrc.gov.uk	HM Revenue and Customs	HMRC
www.housingcorp.gov.uk	Housing Corporation	
www.inbiz.co.uk	InBiz	
www.employmenttribunalsni.co.uk	Industrial Tribunals and the Fair Employment Tribunal (Northern Ireland)	
www.icg-uk.org	Institute of Career Guidance	ICG
www.ilo.org	International Labour Organization? check	ILO
www.investni.com	Invest Northern Ireland	
www.j4b.com	j4b plc	

www.gov.je	Jersey Government	
www.jobbrokersearch.gov.uk	Job Broker Search	
www.jobcentreplus.gov.uk	Jobcentre Plus	
www.jfo.org.uk	Just Fight On!	
www.lra.org.uk	Labour Relations Agency Northern Ireland	
www.learndirect.co.uk	Learndirect	
www.lsc.gov.uk	Learning and Skills Council	LSC
www.lampdirect.org.uk	Leicestershire Action for Mental Health Project	LAMP
www.leonard-cheshire.org	Leonard Cheshire Foundation	
www.lifelonglearninguk.org	Lifelong Learning UK	
www.mencap.org.uk	Mencap	MENCAP
www.mentalhealth.org.uk	Mental Health Foundation	MHF
www.mhrn.info	Mental Health Research Network	MHRN
www.mtm.org	Methods Time Measurement	MTM
www.mind.org.uk	MIND (National Association for Mental Health)	MIND
www.mindfulemployer.net	Mindful Employer	
www.mindtools.com	MindTools	
http://diversity.monster.co.uk	Monster.co.uk: equality and diversity	
www.motability.co.uk	Motability	
www.mssociety.org.uk	Multiple Sclerosis Society	
www.navca.org.uk	National Association for Voluntary and Community Action	NAVCA
www.ncvo-vol.org.uk	National Council for Voluntary Organisations	NCVO
www.ncwe.org	National Council for Workforce Education	NCWE
www.nationaldebtline.co.uk	National Debtline	
www.nebosh.org.uk	National Examination Board in Occupational Safety and Health	NEBOSH
www.nhs.uk	National Health Service England	NHS
www.housing.org.uk	National Housing Federation	NFS
www.nimhe.org.uk	National Institute for Mental Health in England	NIMHE
www.nrac.org.uk	National Register of Access Consultants	NRAC
www.nationalunderwriter.com	National Underwriter Company (USA)	NUCO
www.nddp.com	New Deal for Disabled People	NDDP
www.nhsplus.nhs.uk	NHS Plus	
www.nihe.gov.uk	Northern Ireland Housing Executive	NIHE
www.onetcenter.org	O*NET (Occupational Information Network, USA)	O*NET

www.oscr.org.uk	Office of the Scottish Charity Regulator	OSCR
www.ontheside.org	On the Side	
www.papworth.org.uk	Papworth Trust	
www.pow-bps.com	People and Organisations @ Work	
www.physiofirst.org.uk	Physio First	
www.princes-trust.org.uk	Prince's Trust	
www.poosh.org	Professional Organisations in Occupational Safety and Health	POOSH
www.prospects.ac.uk	Prospects	
www.radar.org.uk	RADAR (Royal Association for Disability and Rehabilitation)	RADAR
www.rec.uk.com	Recruitment and Employment Confederation	REC
www.rehabuk.org	Rehab UK	
www.rehabwindow.net	Rehab Window	
www.rcaa.org.au	Rehabilitation Counselling Association of Australasia	
www.remploy.co.uk	Remploy	
www.roymatheson.com	Roy Matheson Associates	
www.rcn.org.uk	Royal College of Nursing	RCN
www.rcplondon.ac.uk	Royal College of Physicians	RCP
www.rnid.org.uk	Royal National Institute for the Deaf	RNID
www.rnib.org.uk	Royal National Institute of the Blind	RNIB
www.scmh.org.uk	Sainsbury Centre for Mental Health: Employment and Health Innovations Network	SCMH/NEHIN
www.scope.org.uk	Scope	
www.scvo.org.uk	Scottish Council for Voluntary Organisations	SCVO
www.scottish-enterprise.com	Scottish Enterprise	
www.scotland.gov.uk	Scottish Executive	
www.shaw-trust.org.uk	Shaw Trust	
www.sohas co.uk	Sheffield Occupational Health and Advisory Service	SOHAS
www.shelter.org.uk	Shelter	
www.skill.org.uk	Skill	
www.skymark.com	SkyMark	
www.socialexclusionunit.gov.uk	Social Exclusion Unit	
www.socialfirms.co.uk	Social Firms UK	
www.ssa.gov	Social Security Administration (USA)	
www.siop.org	Society for Industrial and Organizational Psychology (USA)	
www.som.org.uk	Society of Occupational Medicine	SOM
www.spinal.co.uk	Spinal Injuries Association	SIA
www.sthkhealth.nhs.uk	St Helens and Knowsley Health Trust	

www.stop-rsi.co.uk	Stop RSI	
www.supply2.gov.uk	Supply2.gov.uk	
www.support-dogs.org.uk	Support Dogs	
http://dms.dartmouth.edu/prc/instruments/model	Supported Employment Fidelity Scale (Dartmouth Psychiatric Research Centre)	
www.surestart.gov.uk	Sure Start	
www.bohs.org	British Occupational Hygiene Society (BOHS)	BOHS
www.csp.org.uk	Chartered Society of Physiotherapy	CSP
www.iosh.co.uk	Institution of Occupational Safety and Health	IOSH
www.som.org.uk	Society of Occupational Medicine	SOM
www.theodora.com	Theodora	
www.tateproject.org.uk	Through Assistive Technology to Employment	TATE
www.tuc.org.uk	Trades Union Congress	TUC
www.employmenttribunals.gov.uk	Tribunals Service: Employment	
www.troubleatwork.org.uk	troubleatwork	
www.bcodp.org.uk	UK Disabled People's Council	UKDPC
www.direct.gov.uk	Direct Gov	
www.ukhca.co.uk	UK Home Care Association	UKHCA
www.unionlearn.org.uk	unionlearn	
www.unison.org.uk	UNISON	
www.unumprovident.co.uk	Unum Provident	
www.valuebasedmanagement.net	Value Based Management	
www.vocationalrehabilitationassociation.org.uk	Vocational Rehabilitation Association	VRA
www.volunteering-ni.org/	Volunteer Development Agency in Northern Ireland	
www.volunteerscotland.org.uk/.	Volunteer Scotland	
www.volunteering.org.uk	Volunteering England	
www.volunteering-wales.net/	Volunteering Wales	
www.wcva.org.uk	Wales Council for Voluntary Action	WCVA
new.wales.gov.uk.	Welsh Assembly	
www.worksupport.com	Work Support	
www.workcover.wa.gov.au	WorkCover (Australia)	
www.workingbacksscotland.com	Working Backs Scotland	
www.workingforhealthni.gov.uk	Working for Health Northern Ireland	
www.whig.org.uk	Workplace and Health Information Gateway	WHIG
www.workplacehealthconnect.co.uk	Workplace Health Connect	WHC
www.yell.com	Yellow Pages	
www.youreable.com	You're Able	

REFERENCES

(all website addresses accessed 7 March 2007)

Accreditation Council on Services for People with Disabilities (1993) *Outcome-based performance measures*. Maryland, USA: Accreditation Council.

Agency for Health Policy and Research (1994) *AHCPR: Guidelines #14, Clinical Practice Guidelines 95-0642*. US Department of Health and Human Services, Public Health Service, December 8.

Arnold D (2005) OTs urged to offer career advice to young disabled. *Therapy Weekly* December 1, p. 4.

Association of British Insurers (2004) *Availability of Rehabilitation Services in the UK*. ABI. (www.abi.org.uk/Bookshop/Archive.asp)

Association of British Insurers (2005) *UK Insurance Key Facts*. ABI. (www.abi.org.uk)

Association of British Insurers (2006) *Care and Good Health: Improving Health in the Workplace*. ABI.

Association of Personal Injury Lawyers (2004) *Best Practice Guide on Rehabilitation*. APIL.

Bandura A (1986) *Social Foundations of Thought and Action: A Social Cognitive Theory*. Engelwood Cliffs, NJ: Prentice Hall.

Bandura A (1995) *Self-Efficacy: The Exercise of Control*. New York: Freeman, p. 382.

Barnes H & Hudson M (2006) *Pathways to Work: Qualitative research on the condition management programme*. Research report No 346. DWP. (www.dwp.gov.uk)

Baronet A-M & Gerber GJ (1998) Psychiatric rehabilitation: efficacy of four models. *Clinical Psychology Review* 18: 189–228.

Beveridge W (1942) *Social Insurance and Allied Services*. London: HMSO.

Blesedell Crepeau E, Cohn ES & Boyt Schell BA (2003) *Willard and Spackman's Occupational Therapy (10th edn)* Philadelphia, PA: Lippincott Williams & Wilkins

Bond GR, Becker DR, Drake RE & Vogler KM (1998) A fidelity scale for the individual placement and support model of supported employment. *Rehabilitation Counseling Bulletin* 40(4): 265–284.

Boyt Schell BA (2003) Clinical reasoning: the basis of practice. In Blesedell Crepeau E, Cohn ES, Boyt Schell BA (2003) *Willard and Spackman's Occupational Therapy (10th edn)* Philadelphia, PA: Lippincott Williams & Wilkins, Ch 11.

Bransford JD & Stein BS (1984) *The IDEAL Problem Solver: A Guide for Improving, Thinking, Learning, and Creativity*. New York: WH Freeman & Company.

Brooker A, Cole DC, Hogg-Johnson S, Smith J & Frank JW (2001) Modified work: prevalence and characteristics in a sample of workers with soft-tissue injuries. *Journal of Occupational and Environmental Medicine* 43: 276–284.

Brown D & Brooks L (1996) *Career choice and Development (3rd edn)*. San Francisco: Jossey Bass.

Burbidge A (2003) Conference Reports: Recent advances in predicting the response to clinical rehabilitation. *Clinical Medicine* 3: 172–175.

Burchardt T (2005) *The Education and Employment of Disabled Young People: Frustrated Ambition.* (Joseph Rowntree Foundation). Bristol: The Policy Press.

Burton A, Main C (2000) Obstacles to recovery from work-related musculoskeletal disorders. In Karwowski W (ed) *International Encyclopedia of Ergonomics and Human Factors.* London: Taylor and Francis.

Butterworth R (2005) *The guiding principles and practice which govern good job retention services.* Sainsbury Centre for Mental Health (www.scmh.org.uk)

Buzan T (no date) *Mind Maps.* Available at www.buzanworld.com/mindmaps

Canelón MF (1995) Job site analysis facilitates work reintegration. *American Journal of Occupational Therapy* 49(5): 461–467.

Carey P, Farrell J, Hui M & Sullivan B (2001) *Heyde's MODAPTS: A language of work.* Sydney, Australia: Heyde Dynamics.

Chambers R, Moore S, Parker G & Slovak A (2001) *Occupational Health Matters in General Practice.* Staffordshire University. Oxford: Radcliffe Medical Press.

Charlton JE (ed) (2005) *Core Curriculum for Professional Education in Pain.* Seattle: IASP Press.

Chartered Institute of Personnel and Development (CIPD) (2006) Incapacity Benefit Reform: Why it is needed and how to engage employers. *Impact* 15: 22–25. (www.cipd.co.uk)

Covey S (1994) *First Things First.* USA: Simon & Schuster, USA.

Cox T, Griffiths A & Rial-Gonzalez E (2000) *Research on Work-Related Stress.* Luxembourg: European Agency for Safety and Health at Work.

Creed PA, Machin MA & Hicks R (1999) Improving mental health status and coping abilities for long term unemployed youth using cognitive behavioural therapy-based interventions. *Journal of Organisational Behaviour* 20: 963–978.

Cromwell FS (1985) *Work-related Programs in Occupational Therapy.* New York: Haworth Press.

Crowther R, Marshall M, Bond G & Huxley P (2004) Vocational rehabilitation for people with severe mental illness (Cochrane Review). *Cochrane Library* Issue 1. Chichester: John Wiley & Sons Ltd. (www.cochrane.org)

Curtis J Origins of vocational rehabilitation as we know it. Rehabwindow (www.rehabwindow.net)

Dannenbaum SE & Shaffer IA (2005) The benefits of group teleconferencing: helping workers with psychiatric disabilities return to work. *Life and Health.* The National Underwriter Company, USA. May 18 (www.nationalunderwriter.com)

Davis A, Pound E & Stafford B (2006) *New Deal For Disabled People Extensions: Examining the Role and Operation of New Job Brokers.* London: Department for Work and Pensions, Research Report No 384. (www.dwp.gov.uk/asd/asd5/rports2005-2006/rrep384.pdf)

de Buck PDM, Schoones JW, Allaire SH & Vliet Vlieland TPM (2002) Vocational rehabilitation in patients with chronic rheumatic diseases: A systematic literature review. *Seminars in Arthritis and Rheumatism* 32: 196–203. Cited in Waddell G, Burton AK & Bartys S (2004)

de Gaudemaris R (2000) Clinical issues: return to work and public safety. *Occupational Medicine: State of the Art Reviews* 15: 223–230. Cited in Waddell G, Burton AK & Bartys S (2004) *Concepts of Rehabilitation for the Management of Common Health Problems.* London: DWP.

de Jonge D, Scherer M & Rodger S (2007) Assistive Technology in the Workplace. Philadelphia: Elsevier.

Department for Education and Skills (2004) *Five Year Strategy for Children and Learners.* London: The Stationery Office.

Department for Education and Skills (2005) *Skills: Getting On In Business, Getting On At Work* White Paper. London: The Stationery Office.

Department of Health (2004) *Choosing Health: Making Healthy Choices Easier.* London: DH.

Department of Health (2006) *Vocational Services for People with Severe Mental Health Problems: Commissioning Guidance.* London: DH.

Department of Work and Pensions (2004a) *Building Capacity for Work: A UK Framework for Vocational Rehabilitation.* London: DWP.

Department of Work and Pensions (2004b) *Employers Liability Compulsory Insurance Review.* London: DWP.

Department of Work and Pensions, Department of Health, Health and Safety Executive (2005) *Health, Work and Well-being: Caring for our Future.* London: DWP.

Devereux J (2003) Work-related stress as a risk factor for WMSDs: implications for ergonomics interventions. In McCabe PT (ed) *Contemporary Ergonomics* pp. 59–64, London: Taylor & Francis.

Devlin C, Burnside L & Akroyd L (2006) Mental health vocational rehabilitation: an overview of occupational therapy service provision in Northern Ireland. *British Journal of Occupational Therapy* 69(7): 334–338.

Dionne CE (1999) Low back pain. In Crombie I, Croft P, Linton S, Le Resche L & Von Korff M (eds) *Epidemiology of Pain.* Seattle: IASP Press.

Disability Employment Coalition (2004) *Access to Work for Disabled People.* London: RNIB.

Ellexson MT (1997) Job analysis. In American Occupational Therapy Association (AOTA) (1997) *Work: Principles and Practice.* AOTA.

Engel G (1977) The need for a new medical model: challenge for biomedicine. *Journal of Science* 196: 129–136.

Enright MS (1996) The relationship between disability status, career beliefs and career indecision. *Rehabilitation Counseling Bulletin* 40(2): 134–152.

Fairbank JC, Couper J, Davies JB & O'Brien JP (1980) The Oswestry low back pain disability questionnaire. *Physiotherapy* 66(8): 271–273.

Farrell J & Littlejohn G (1999) Pain, nature of task, and body part used in fibromyalgia syndrome. *Journal of Musculoskeletal Pain* 7(1/2): 279–284.

Feuerstein M, Marshall L, Shaw WS & Burrell LM (2000) Multicomponent intervention for work-related upper extremity disorders. *Journal of Occupational Rehabilitation* 10(1): 71–83.

Fleishman E & Mumford M (1991) Evaluation classifications of job behaviour: A construct validation of the ability requirement scales. *Personnel Psychology* 44: 522–575.

Floyd M (ed) (1997) *Vocational Rehabilitation and Europe.* London: Jessica Kingsley.

Floyd M (2002) *Vocational Rehabilitation in the UK*: Institute for Public Policy Research Seminar. London: Rehabilitation Resource Centre, City University.

Floyd M & Barrett (2005) Vocational rehabilitation policies and programmes: what can we learn from other countries? *Work* 24: 117–122.

Frank JW, Brooker A-S, DeMaio SE, Kerr MS, Maetzel A, Shannon HS, Sullivan TJ, Norman RW & Wells RP (1996) Disability resulting from occupational low back pain. Part II: What do we know about secondary prevention? A review of the scientific evidence on prevention after disability begins. *Spine* 21: 2918–2929.

Frank J, Sinclair S, Hogg-Johnson S, Shannon H, Bombardier C, Beaton D & Cole D (1998) Preventing disability from work-related low-back pain. New evidence gives new hope –

if we can just get all the players onside. *Canadian Medical Association Journal* 158: 1625–1631.

French Gilson S (1998) Case management and supported employment: a good fit. *Journal of Case Management* 7(1): 10–17.

Frost P & Reel K (2006) New opportunities with pathways to work. *OT News* September 30.

Ghates LB (2000) Workplace accommodation as a social process. *Journal of Occupational Rehabilitation* 10: 85–97.

Gibson L & Strong J (2003) An Occupational Therapy framework of functional capacity evaluation in work rehabilitation. *Australian Journal of Occupational Therapy* 50: 64–71

Gilworth G, Chamberlain MA, Harvey A, Woodhouse A, Smith J, Smyth MG & Tennant A (2003) Development of a work instability scale for rheumatoid arthritis. *Arthritis Care and Research* 49(3): 349–354.

Godby S (2005, unpublished) The Occupational Therapy contribution to vocational rehabilitation. College of Occupational Therapists Specialist Section OTWPP, Symposium 25 November 2005.

Grbich C (1999) *Qualitative Research in Health: an Introduction.* Thousand Oaks, CA: Sage Publications.

Grove B (2005) *Condition Management Programmes. Economic Inactivity and Ill Health*: Challenges and Solutions Event, Cardiff, November 2005.

Hagedorn R (2000) *Tools for Practice in Occupational Therapy: A Structured Approach to Core Skills.* Edinburgh: Churchill Livingstone.

Hagner D, Noll A & Enein-Donovan L (2002) Identifying community employment program staff competencies: A critical incident approach. *Journal of Rehabilitation* 68(1): 45–51.

Haldorson EMH, Grasdal AL, Skouen JS, Risa AE, Kronholm K & Ursin H (2002) Higher RTW rates can be achieved for workers with musculoskeletal pain who have medium or poor prognosis for RTW if they receive light or extensive multidisciplinary treatments, respectively. *Pain* 95: 49–63.

Handy C (1993) *Understanding Organisations (4th edn).* Harmondsworth: Penguin.

Hansen AJ, Edlund C & Henningsson M (2004) Factors relevant to a return to work: A multivariate approach. *Work* 26: 179–190.

Health and Safety Commission (1974) *The Health and Safety at Work Act.* London: HMSO.

Health and Safety Commission (2000) *Securing Health Together. A Long-term Occupational Health Strategy for England Scotland and Wales.* London: HSE Books.

Health and Safety Commission (2004) *Strategy for Workplace Health and Safety in Great Britain to 2010.* London: HSE Books.

Health and Safety Executive (2003) *Work with Display Screen Equipment. Guidance on Regulations.* London: HSE Books, L26.

Health and Safety Executive (2004) *Managing Sickness Absence And Return To Work: An Employers' And Managers' Guide.* London: HSE Books, HSG249.

Health and Safety Executive (2005a) *Obstacles to Recovery from Musculoskeletal Disorder In Industry.* (www.hse.gov.uk/research/rrpdf/rr323.pdf)

Health and Safety Executive (2005b) *Working Together to Prevent Sickness Absence Becoming Job Loss.* HSE, WEB02. (www.hse.gov.uk/pubns/web02.pdf)

Hershenson (1996) Work Adjustment: a neglected area in career counseling. *Journal of Counseling and Development* 74: 442–446.

House of Commons Select Committee on Work and Pensions (July 2004) 4th Report. (www.publications.parliament.uk/pa/cm200304/cmselect/cmworpen/456/45602.htm)

Howard A (1995) *The Changing Nature Of Work*. San Francisco, CA: Jossey-Bass.

Huang YH, Pransky GS, Shaw WS, Benjamin KL, Savageau JA (2006) Factors affecting the organizational responses of employers to workers with injuries. *Work* 26: 75–84.

Ilmarinen J (2003) *Work Ability Index: A Tool for Occupational Health Research and Practice*. Finnish Institute of Occupational Health. (www.bgf-tagung.ch/Symposien/ Workability_e_Index.pdf)

Inge KJ (2006) Assistive technology as a workplace support. *Journal of Vocational Rehabilitation* 24: 67–71.

Innes E & Straker L (2002) Strategies used when conducting work-related assessments. *Work* 19: 149–165.

Inman J, McGurk E, Smith J et al. (2005/06) Is vocational rehabilitation a transition to recovery for individuals with severe and enduring mental health problems? *Public Involvement in Health Research in the North West, Report of the Success Stories Mapping Project and Conference 2005/6*. North West User Research Advisory Group in conjunction with Health R&D North West.

Institute for Work and Health, American Academy of Orthopedic Surgeons (1996) *Disabilities of the Arm, Shoulder and Hand (DASH) Outcome Measure*. Institute for Work and Health. (www.dash.iwh.on.ca/conditions.htm)

Isernhagen SJ (2000) Primary and secondary therapy for the acute musculoskeletal disorder. In Mayer TG, Gatchel RJ & Polatin PB (eds) *Occupational Musculoskeletal Disorders: Function, Outcomes and Evidence*. Philadelphia, PA: Lippincott Williams & Wilkins, pp. 323–338.

Jacobs K (1991) *Occupational Therapy: Work-related Programs and Assessments (2nd edn)*. London: Little, Brown & Co.

Japp J (2005) *Brain Injury and Returning to Employment: A Guide for Practitioners*. London: Jessica Kingsley.

Karsh BT, Moro FBP & Smith MJ (2001) The efficacy of workplace ergonomic interventions to control musculoskeletal disorders: a critical analysis of the peer-reviewed literature. *Theoretical Issues in Ergonomic Science* 2: 23–96. Cited in Waddell G, Burton AK & Bartys S (2004) *Concepts of Rehabilitation for the Management of Common Health Problems*. London: DWP.

Kendall N, Linton S & Main C (1997) *Guide to Assessing Psychosocial Yellow Flags in Acute Low Back Pain: Risk Factors for Long Term Disability and Work Loss*. New Zealand: Accident and Rehabilitation and Compensation Insurance Corporation of New Zealand and the National Health Committee.

Kielhofner G (1980). A model of human occupation, part two. Ontogenesis from the perspective of temporal adaptation. *American Journal of Occupational Therapy* 34: 657–663.

Kirsh B (2006) Commentary. *International Journal of Therapy and Rehabilitation* 13(3): 134.

Krause N, Dasinger LK & Neuhauser F (1998) Modified work and return to work: a review of the literature. *Journal of Occupational Rehabilitation* 8: 113–139.

Langford R (2005) A rehabilitation and retention service in an NHS occupational health setting. *Occupational Therapy in Work: Practice and Productivity Newsletter* 70: 13–15.

Law M, Baptiste S, Carswell A, McColl MA. Polatajko H & Pollock N (1998) *Canadian Occupational Performance Measure*. Ottawa: Canadian Association of Occupational Therapists.

Lawlis GF, Cuencas R, Selby D, et al. (1989) The development of the Dallas Pain Questionnaire for illness behaviour. *Spine* 14: 511.

Leach S (2002) *A Supported Employment Workbook*. London: Jessica Kingsley.

Locke EA & Latham GP (2002) Building a practically useful theory of goal setting and task motivation. *American Psychologist* 57(9): 705–717.

Macdonald H (2004 unpublished) *Cognitive–Behavioural Psychotherapy in Return to Work Programmes*. OTWPP Symposium 2004, handout.

Machin A & Creed P (1999) *Changing Wonky Beliefs Program*. (www.usq.edu.au/users/machin/cwb.htm)

Main CJ & Burton AK (1998) Pain mechanisms. In McCaig R & Harrington M (eds) *The Changing Face of Occupational Health*. London: Health & Safety Executive, pp. 233–253.

Main CJ & Burton AK (2000) Economic and occupational influences on pain and disability. In Main CJ & Spanswick CC (eds) *Pain Management: An Interdisciplinary Approach*. Edinburgh: Churchill Livingstone.

Main L & Haig J (2006) Occupational therapy and vocational rehabilitation: an audit of an outpatient occupational therapy service. *British Journal of Occupational Therapy* 69(6): 288–292.

Maitland I (1999) *Managing Your Time*. London: Chartered Institute of Personnel and Development.

Marchington M & Wilkinson A (2003) *People Management and Development: Human Resource Management at Work (2nd edn)*. London: Chartered Institute of Personnel and Development.

Matheson LN (1993) *Physical Demand Characteristics Of Work*. USA: Department of Labor.

Matheson R (2002) *Work Hardening Course*. Roy Matheson Associates, Inc., USA. (www.roymatheson.com)

Matheson R (2004) *The Functional Capacity Evaluation Certification Program* Chapter 9. Roy Matheson Associates, Inc., USA. (www.roymatheson.com)

Mattingly C (1998) *Healing Dramas and Clinical Plots: The Narrative Structure of Experience*. Cambridge: Cambridge University Press.

McCue M, Pramuka M, Chase S & Fabry P (1994) Functional assessment procedures for individuals with severe cognitive disorders. *American Rehabilitation* Autumn 1994.

McDonald R (1996–97) *Career Decision Making: Opposing Views*. Graduate Diploma of career development. Deaking University, Melbourne, Australia.

Melzack R (1975) The McGill Pain Questionnaire: major properties and scoring methods. *Pain* 1: 277–299.

Menz FE, Botterbusch K, HagenFoley D & Johnson PT (2003) Achieving quality outcomes through community-based rehabilitation programmes: the results are in. Presented to NISH National Training Conference, April 7, Denver, Colorado. Cited in Waddell G, Burton AK & Bartys S (2004) *Concepts of Rehabilitation for the Management of Common Health Problems*. London: DWP.

Miller AR, Treiman DJ, Cain PS & Roos PA (1980) *Work, Jobs, and Occupations: A Critical Review of the Dictionary of Occupational Titles, Commission on Behavioral and Social Sciences and Education*. Washington DC: National Academy Press.

Mind Tools Ltd (2006) *The Mind Tools e-book*. (www.mindtools.com)

Mindout (2002) *Working Minds Toolkit: A Practical Resource to Promote Good Workplace Practice on Mental Health*. (http://kc.nimhe.org.uk/upload/Working%20Minds%20Toolkit.pdf)

Mindout (2003) *Line Managers' Resource: A Practical Guide to Managing and Supporting Mental Health in the Workplace*. (www.mindfulemployer.net)

Mital A & Mital A (2002) Returning coronary heart disease patients to work: A modified perspective. *Journal of Occupational Rehabilitation* 12: 31–42.

Monninkhof EM, van der Valk PDLPM, van der Palen J, van Herwaarden CLA, Partridge MR, Walters EH & Zielhuis GA (2003) Self-management education for chronic obstructive pulmonary disease (Cochrane Review). In *The Cochrane Library*, Issue 4. Chichester: John Wiley & Sons Ltd.

Moore-Corner RA, Kielfhofner G & Olson L (1998) *Work Environment Impact Scale (WEIS) version 2.0*. Model of Human Occupation Clearing House, University of Illinois, USA.

Nadeau B & Buckheit C (1995) Work simulation as a diagnostic tool in the rehabilitation setting. *Occupational Therapy in Health Care* 9(1): 37–44.

Neenan M & Dryden W (2002) *Life Coaching: A Cognitive Behavioural Approach*. Hove: Brunner and Routledge.

Nordqvist C, Holmqvist C & Alexanderson K (2003) Views of laypersons on the role employers play in return to work when sick-listed. *Journal of Occupational Rehabilitation* 13: 11–20.

Norman G (2005) Research in clinical reasoning: Past history and current trends. *Medical Education* 39(4): 418–427.

Northern Ireland Committee of the College of Occupational Therapists (1992) *Employment Assessment and Preparation in Occupational Therapy*. College of Occupational Therapists.

Olsheski JA, Rosenthal DA & Hamilton M (2002) Disability management and psychosocial rehabilitation: Considerations for integration. *Work* 19: 63–70.

Paley J, Eva G & Duncan E (2006) In-order-to analysis: an alternative to classifying different levels of occupational activity. *British Journal of Occupational Therapy* 69(4): 161–168.

Palmer G, Carr J & Kenway P (2006) *Monitoring Poverty and Social Exclusion*. York: Joseph Rowntree Foundation.

Perry D (2001) *Vocational Rehabilitation and Employment: From Principles to Practice*. Technical Background Paper. ILO-EASMAT. (www.ilo.org)

Pransky G, Robertson MM & Moon SD (2002) Stress and work-related upper extremity disorders: implications for prevention and management. *American Journal of Industrial Medicine* 41: 443–455.

Pransky GS, Shaw WS, Franche R-L & Clarke A (2004) Disability prevention and communication among workers, physicians, employers, and insurers – current models and opportunities for improvement. *Disability & Rehabilitation* 26(11): 625–634.

Pratt J & Jacobs K (1997) Work Practice: International Perspectives. Oxford: Butterworth Heinemann.

Punch R, Creed PA & Hyde M (2005) Predicting career development in hard-of-hearing adolescents in Australia. *Journal of Deaf Studies and Deaf Education* 10(2): 146–160.

Raptosh D (2005) *Functional Capacity Evaluation*. The Bureau of Workers' Compensation. 4th Annual Workers' Compensation Conference Handout. (www.dli.state.pa.us/landi/cwp/view.asp?A=138&Q=222715&tx=1)

Rehab UK (2005) *The Brain Injury Handbook*. London: Rehab UK. (www.rehabuk.org)

Reidy-Croft S (online) *Factors Impacting Successful Return to Work: Identifying Potential Long-Term, High Cost Claims*. Australia: Work Cover (www.workcover.wa.gov.au)

Rinaldi M, Perkins R, Hardisty J, Harding E, Taylor A & Brown S (2004) Implementing a user employment programme in a mental health trust – lessons learned. *A Life in the Day* 8(4): 9–14.

Robdale N (2005) Stepping in early: a job retention scheme. *A Life in the Day* 9(1).

Roulstone A & Barnes C (2005) *Working Futures: Disabled People, Policy and Social Inclusion*. Bristol: The Policy Press.

Rubin RS (2002) *Will the real SMART goals please stand up?* Society for Industrial and Organizational Psychology Inc., USA. (www.siop.org)

Sandqvist J, Henriksson C (2004) Work functioning: a conceptual framework. *Work* 23: 147–157.

Savickas M & Lent R (1994) Convergence in career development theories. California: Consulting Psychologists Press Inc. (www.extension.psu.edu/workforce/Briefs/OverviewCareerDev(Insert).pdf)

Schonstein E, Kenny DT, Keating J & Koes BW (2002) *Work Conditioning, Work Hardening and Functional Restoration for Workers With Back and Neck Pain*. (Cochrane Review). *Cochrane Library* Issue 1. Chichester: John Wiley & Sons Ltd. (www.cochrane.org)

Sharf RS (1992) *Applying Career Development Theory to Counselling*. California: Brooks/Cole.

Shaw KL, Hackett J, Southwood TR & McDonagh JE (2006) The prevocational and early employment needs of adolescents with juvenile idiopathic arthritis: the adolescent perspective. *British Journal of Occupational Therapy* 69(3): 98–105.

Shaw L, Segal R, Polatajko H & Harburn K (2002) Understanding return to work behaviours: promoting the importance of individual perceptions in the study of return to work. *Disability and Rehabilitation* 24(4): 185–195.

Shaw WS, Robertson MM & McLellan RK (2003) Employee perspectives on the role of supervisors to prevent workplace disability after injuries. *Journal of Occupational Rehabilitation* 13: 129–142.

Shaw WS, Robertson MM, Pransky G, McLellan RK & Strasser PB (2006) Training to optimize the response of supervisors to work injuries – needs assessment, design, and evaluation. *American Association of Occupational Health Nursing Journal* 54(5): 226–235.

Skinner NJ (2002) The role of goal setting in workforce development. In Roche AM & McDonald J (eds) *Catching Clouds. Exploring Workforce Development for the Alcohol and Other Drugs Field*. Adelaide, Australia: National Centre for Education and Training on Addiction, Flinders University. (www.nceta.flinders.edu.au/pdf/proceedings2002/skinner.pdf)

SkyMark Corporation (2006) *Force Field Diagrams*. (www.skymark.com)

Social Exclusion Unit (2006) *What is Social Exclusion?* (www.socialexclusionunit.gov.uk)

Social Security Online *Mental Residual Functional Capacity Assessment* (Form SSA-4734-F4-SUP) (www.ssa.gov)

Stephenson RC (2004) Using a complexity model of human behaviour to help interprofessional clinical reasoning. *International Journal of Therapy and Rehabilitation* 11(4): 168–175.

Steward B (1997) Employment in the next millennium: the impact of changes in work on health and rehabilitation. *British Journal of Occupational Therapy* 60(6): 268–272.

Stewart L & Wheeler K (2005) Occupation for recovery. *OT News* November: 24–25.

Strauser DR, Ketz K & Keim J (2002) The relationship between self-efficacy, locus of control and work personality – self efficacy and locus of control. *Journal of Rehabilitation* Jan–March.

Stuckey R (1997) Enhancing work performance in industrial settings: a role for occupational therapy. *British Journal of Occupational Therapy* 60(6): 277–278.

Stuckey R & Meyer R (2000) *Workplace Ergonomics for Health Professionals*. Personal communication.

Thomas T, Secker J & Grove B (2002) *The Development of a New Type of Partnership: Promoting Prevention and Retention Issues for Employees With Mental Health Problems*. London: King's College London.

Thomson L, Neathey F & Rick J (2003) *Best Practice in Rehabilitating Employees Following Absence Due To Work-Related Stress*. HSE Research Report 138. London: HSE Books.

Trades Union Congress (2000) *Getting Better At Getting Back*. TUC consultation document on rehabilitation. (www.tuc.org.uk)

Trades Union Congress (2006a) *Disability and Work: A Trade Union Guide to the Law and Good Practice*. (www.tuc.org.uk)

Trades Union Congress (2006b) *Jobs for Disabled People and a Three Point Plan*. (www.tuc.org.uk)

Turk DC & Melzack R (1992) *Handbook of Pain Assessment*. New York: Guilford Press.

Turner E, Barcus MJ, West M & Revell G (unknown date) Personal assistance services: a vital workplace support. The Rehabilitation Research and Training Center at Virginia Commonwealth University. Article 11: 151–160. (www.worksupport.com/resources/listContent.cfm/16/0)

UK Home Care Association (2003) UKHCA Costs calculator for home care version (www.ukhca.co.uk/projectdetails.aspx?projectcode=7)

Unsworth CA (2005) Using a head-mounted video camera to explore current conceptualizations of clinical reasoning in occupational therapy. *American Journal of Occupational Therapy* 59(1): 31–40.

Value Based Management.net (2006) *Force Field Analysis* – Lewin, Kurt (www.valuebasedmanagement.net)

van der Klink JJL & van Dijk FJH (2003) Dutch practice guidelines for managing adjustment disorders in occupational and primary health care. *Scandinavian Journal of Work and Environmental Health* 29: 478–487. Cited in Waddell G, Burton AK & Bartys S (2004) *Concepts of Rehabilitation for the Management Of Common Health Problems*. London: DWP.

van Tulder M & Koes B (2002) Low back pain and sciatica (chronic). *Clinical Evidence* 7: 1032–1048. Cited in Waddell G, Burton AK & Bartys S (2004) *Concepts of Rehabilitation for the Management Of Common Health Problems*. London: DWP.

Velozo C, Kielhofner G & Fisher G (1998) *A User's Guide to Worker Role Interview (WRI)* version 9.0. Model of Human Occupation Clearing House, University of Illinois, USA.

Vernon H & Mior S (1991) The Neck Disability Index: a study of reliability and validity. *Journal of Manipulative and Physiological Therapeutics* 14(7): 409–415.

Vinokur AD & Schul Y (2002) The web of coping resources and pathways to re-employment following a job loss. *Journal of Occupational Health Psychology* 7(1): 68–83.

Vinokur AD, Schul Y, Vuori J & Price RH (2000) Two years after a job loss: long-term impact of the JOBS program on reemployment and mental health. *Journal of Occupational Health Psychology* 5(1): 32–47.

Vocational Rehabilitation Association (2006) *Recognising and Accrediting Education and Training Provision for the Vocational Rehabilitation Professional. The Way Forward*: A consultation paper. Glasgow: VRA.

Waddell G & Aylward M (2005) *The Scientific and Conceptual Basis of Incapacity Benefits*. London: The Stationery Office.

Waddell G & Burton AK (2000) *Occupational Health Guidelines for the Management of Low Back Pain At Work*. London: Faculty of Occupational Medicine.

Waddell G & Watson PJ (2004) Rehabilitation. In Waddell G (ed) *The Back Pain Revolution (2nd edn)*. Edinburgh: Churchill Livingstone.

Waddell G, Burton AK & Main CJ (2003) *Screening for Risk of Long-term Incapacity: A Conceptual and Scientific Review*. London: The Royal Society of Medicine Press.

Waddell G, Burton AK & Bartys S (2004) *Concepts of Rehabilitation for the Management of Common Health Problems*. Evidence base available at http://www.dwp.gov.uk/medical/publications/rehab-appendices/

Woodruffe C (1992) In Marchington, M & Wilkinson, A (2003) *People Management and Development: Human Resource Management at Work*. London: Chartered Institute of Personnel and Development.

World Health Organization (1974) cited in Hagedorn R (1992) *Occupational Therapy: Foundations for Practice*. Edinburgh: Churchill Livingstone.

World Health Organization (2002) *International Classification of Functioning, Disability and Health*. WHO Workplace and Health Information Gateway (WHIG). (www.whig.org.uk)

Wright M, Bearsden C & Marsden S (2004) *Availability of Rehabilitation Services in the UK: A Research Study for the Association of British Insurers*. Reading: Greenstreet Berman Ltd. (www.abi.org.uk)

Zandin Kjell B (2003) *MOST Work Measurement Systems*. USA: Marcel Dekker Inc.

INDEX